The
Antidepressant Solution

A Step-by-Step Guide to Safely
Overcoming Antidepressant Withdrawal,
Dependence, and "Addiction"

JOSEPH GLENMULLEN, M.D.

Free Press
New York London Toronto Sydney

To Ciara, Peter, and Michael

This publication contains the opinions and ideas of its author. It is intended to provide helpful and informative material on the subjects addressed in the publication. It is sold with the understanding that the author and publisher are not engaged in rendering medical, health, or any other kind of personal professional services in the book. The reader should consult his or her medical, health, or other competent professional before adopting any of the suggestions in this book or drawing inferences from it.

The author and publisher specifically disclaim all responsibility for any liability, loss, or risk, personal or otherwise, which is incurred as a consequence, directly or indirectly, of the use and application of any of the contents of this book.

While the case studies described in this book are based on interviews with real persons, including patients treated by the author, the names, professions, locations, and other biographical details about the participants have been changed.

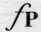
FREE PRESS
A Division of Simon & Schuster, Inc.
1230 Avenue of the Americas
New York, NY 10020

First Free Press trade paperback edition 2006

FREE PRESS and colophon are trademarks of Simon & Schuster, Inc.

For information about special discounts for bulk purchases,
please contact Simon & Schuster Special Sales:
1-800-456-6798 or business@simonandschuster.com

Designed by Paul Dippolito

Manufactured in the United States of America

10 9 8 7 6 5 3 4 2 1

The Library of Congress has catalogued the hardcover edition as follows:
Glenmullen, Joseph.
The antidepressant solution: a step-by-step guide to safely overcoming antidepressant withdrawal, dependence, and "addiction" / Joseph Glenmullen.
p. cm.
Includes bibliographical references and index.
1. Antidepressants. I. Title.
RM332.G56 2005
616.85'27061—dc22   2004063202

ISBN-13: 978-0-7432-6972-8   ISBN-13: 978-0-7432-6973-5 (Pbk)
ISBN-10:   0-7432-6972-1   ISBN-10:   0-7432-6973-X (Pbk)

CONTENTS

PREFACE

As I wrote this book in 2004, doctors and the public experienced an up-heaval in their view of the safety of today's popular antidepressants be-cause the Food and Drug Administration issued a pair of warnings that have been startling to many: Antidepressants may make patients suicidal. In the initial March 2004 warning, the FDA asserted that "adult and pe-diatric patients" on antidepressants can develop a range of side effects that may make them suicidal, including "anxiety, agitation, panic attacks, insomnia, irritability, hostility, impulsivity, akathisia (severe restless-ness), hypomania, and mania."[1] The FDA warned that patients may be vulnerable to this lethal side effect "especially at the beginning of therapy or when the dose either increases or decreases," that is, whenever the dose *changes.* Since decreasing the dose of an antidepressant may make patients suicidal, the warning is directly relevant to the subject of this book: how to taper off antidepressants safely and comfortably once one no longer needs them. In the second, October 2004 warning, the FDA upgraded the alert for children and adolescents to the strongest level possible: a prominent black box warning in the official information on the drugs.[2] Said the FDA's director of the office of medical policy, Dr. Robert Temple: "I think we now all believe there is an increase in suicidal thinking and action that is consistent across all the drugs."[3]

The FDA warning is truly historic; it is the first time the agency has acknowledged that antidepressant drugs can make some patients suicidal. Until 2004, the FDA and pharmaceutical industry insisted that suicidal-ity was more likely to be due to a patient's underlying psychiatric condi-tion. Now the FDA has said unequivocally that antidepressant-induced suicidality "is beyond the suicidality as a result of the disease."[4] The FDA warnings apply to all of today's popular antidepressants: Prozac, Zoloft, Paxil, Celexa, Lexapro, Effexor, Cymbalta, Wellbutrin, Remeron, Luvox, and Serzone.[5] Indeed, the warnings apply to all thirty-two antide-pressants currently on the market, including all of the older tricyclic and monoamine oxidase inhibitor antidepressants. The complete list of anti-depressants can be found in Table P.1. In light of the FDA warnings, patients and their doctors should not change the dose of antidepressants up or down without being well informed about how to do so safely and comfortably.

The FDA is following the lead taken by its British counterpart, the Medicines and Healthcare products Regulatory Agency, the MHRA. In 2003, the British issued a series of warnings and virtually banned many antidepressants for children and adolescents under the age of eighteen.[6] The British advised against the drugs because of the evidence in pharmaceutical company studies that the antidepressants are no more effective in children than placebo (dummy) pills but can make children agitated, sleepless, hostile, aggressive, and suicidal. While the British MHRA has virtually banned many antidepressants for some age groups, the FDA warnings have not banned any of the drugs.

The American and British warnings have been accompanied by allegations that the pharmaceutical industry suppressed data on these lethal side effects for years. According to an article in the March 2004 issue of the *Canadian Medical Association Journal*, GlaxoSmithKline tested its drug Paxil on children and adolescents from 1993 to 1996.[7] The article

Table P.1. ANTIDEPRESSANTS COVERED BY THE FDA'S WARNINGS THAT THE DRUGS MAY MAKE PATIENTS SUICIDAL

(Brand names are capitalized; generic names are in parentheses.)

Anafranil (clomipramine)	Paxil (paroxetine)
Aventyl (nortriptyline)	Pexeva (paroxetine mesylate)
Celexa (citalopram)	Prozac (fluoxetine)
Cymbalta (duloxtine)	Remeron (mirtazapine)
Desyrel (trazodone)	Sarafem (fluoxetine)
Effexor (venlafaxine)	Serzone (nefazodone)
Elavil (amitriptyline)	Sinequan (doxepin)
Lexapro (escitalopram)	Surmontil (trimipramine)
Limbitrol (amitriptyline/ chlordiazepoxide)	Symbyax (fluoxetine/olanzapine)
Ludiomil (maprotiline)	Tofranil (imipramine)
Luvox (fluvoxamine)	Tofranil PM (imipramine)
Marplan (isocarboxazid)	Triavil (amitriptyline/ perphenazine)
Nardil (phenelzine)	Vivactil (protriptyline)
Norpramin (desipramine)	Wellbutrin (bupropion)
Pamelor (nortriptyline)	Zoloft (sertraline)
Parnate (tranylcypromine)	Zyban (bupropion)

quotes a secret, internal GlaxoSmithKline report dating to October 1998 saying the studies showed Paxil "failed" to be more effective than placebo pills in depressed children.[8] The secret memorandum urged company executives "to effectively manage the dissemination of these data in order to minimise any potential negative commercial impact" that might "undermine the profile" of Paxil. In other words, the position paper raised concerns that the damaging information might affect Paxil's global sales, which now approach $5 billion a year.[9] How did the report propose to "effectively manage" the potentially damaging results? By selectively publishing the few "positive data" that would appear to make Paxil look good.

To accomplish this goal, GlaxoSmithKline turned to the psychiatrists who conducted the studies for the company. Headed by Dr. Martin Keller, chairman of the Department of Psychiatry and Human Behavior at the Brown University School of Medicine, a group of more than twenty leading academic psychiatrists published the selected Paxil data in the July 2001 issue of the *Journal of the American Academy of Child and Adolescent Psychiatry*.[10] In stark contrast to the 1998 secret, internal GlaxoSmithKline memo, Keller and his colleagues used highly selected pieces of positive data to glowingly conclude in 2001: "Paxil is generally well tolerated and effective for major depression in adolescents."[11]

After the British and FDA warnings, in April 2004 the prestigious medical journal *The Lancet* published a damning critique of Keller's and a number of other similar antidepressant studies.[12] In an accompanying editorial, *The Lancet* expressed outrage over the GlaxoSmithKline internal memo and misleading academic reports.[13] *The Lancet* described the "selective reporting of favourable research" when side effects as serious as drug-induced suicide are at stake as a "catastrophe" that "should be unimaginable." *The Lancet* called the false reassurances of the pharmaceutical industry and the academic psychiatrists who work closely with the industry "an abuse of the trust patients place in their physicians." Calling the burgeoning antidepressant scandal "a disaster," *The Lancet* called for "legal powers" to force pharmaceutical companies to make unpublished data public. Indeed, a growing chorus of consumer advocates and professional organizations, including the American Medical Association, is calling for a public database that lists all pharmaceutical company data from unpublished as well as published studies.[14]

Keller's misleading 2001 report in the *Journal of the American Academy of Child and Adolescent Psychiatry* was highly influential and widely used to promote prescribing antidepressants to children. Since then the use of the drugs for children has skyrocketed.[15] But two years later, in June 2003, the British declared that the data showed Paxil is not effective for depressed children and, in fact, makes them suicidal and aggressive. Immediately following the British announcement, Glaxo-SmithKline sent a "Dear Doctor" letter to physicians in England saying that Paxil should not be prescribed to children under eighteen years of age because it "failed" to work any better than placebo and frequently caused "hostility, agitation, [and] emotional lability (including crying, mood fluctuations, self-harm, suicidal thoughts and attempted suicide)."[16] In June 2004, Eliot Spitzer, the attorney general for the State of New York, filed suit against GlaxoSmithKline charging the company with "fraud" for misrepresenting its studies of Paxil in children.[17] The company ultimately settled the lawsuit and agreed to post both positive and negative drug research results on its website.[18] Psychiatrists like Keller can each make millions of dollars consulting to pharmaceutical companies and have been criticized for "distorted and unbalanced" reporting of studies in "an attempt to show the drug in the most favourable light."[19]

In many instances, pharmaceutical companies ghostwrite the favorable drug studies published in academic journals.[20] In some instances, the psychiatrists may allow companies to put their names on the reports without even seeing all the data.[21] This practice, too, is increasingly coming under fire.

The FDA has been heavily criticized for its handling of antidepressant-induced suicidality.[22] In 2004, the FDA originally suppressed an analysis of the data on children taking antidepressants by their own internal reviewer, Dr. Andrew Mosholder, who concluded that the drugs made children suicidal, much as the British concluded. The Mosholder report was ultimately leaked to the media.[23] In a controversial move, the FDA wasted valuable time and taxpayer dollars having researchers at Columbia University reanalyze the data. The researchers essentially came to the same conclusions Mosholder and the British had.[24] Critics charge that the FDA's investigation of the antidepressant scandal is a conflict of interest since the agency's own reputation is at stake for having approved the drugs in the first place and having swept under the carpet repeated reports of their side effects, including antidepressant-induced suicidality, for over a decade.[25] Critics also point to the revolving door of FDA officials in and out of working for pharmaceutical companies.[26] As

I finish writing this book, several congressmen have opened investigations into the FDA's mishandling of antidepressant side effects.[27] The continuing revelations in the antidepressant scandal have shaken public confidence not only in the drugs but also in the drug companies, academic researchers, and even the FDA.[28]

What do doctors and patients do when patients are ready to go off the drugs if stopping antidepressants abruptly can cause severe withdrawal reactions that include suicidality, impulsivity, aggression, dizziness, vertigo, nausea, vomiting, headaches, tremors, electric "zap" sensations in the brain, anxiety, crying spells, and insomnia? The problem is compounded by the fact that nowadays 70 percent of prescriptions for antidepressants are written by family doctors, many of whom do not know how to taper patients off the drugs.[29] Family doctors are not responsible for the current situation; they have been pressured by HMOs and insurance companies to prescribe antidepressants rather than refer patients to specialists. In a study sponsored by the Robert Wood Johnson Foundation, 72 percent of family doctors expressed frustration over the lack of access to quality mental health services for their patients.[30] Many family doctors are not comfortable writing so many prescriptions for antidepressants, but feel they have little choice in the matter. Most family doctors do not feel they have the background or training to taper patients off the drugs. Even some psychiatrists are unaware of how to taper patients carefully off today's antidepressants. An estimated 20 million people are on antidepressants in this country, including one million children.[31] With so many people using the drugs, withdrawal and dependence have become major problems.

This book is a natural outgrowth of my work as a psychiatrist and educator. I testified as an expert at the FDA hearing that resulted in the historic spring 2004 warning.[32] My last book, *Prozac Backlash: Overcoming the Dangers of Prozac, Zoloft, Paxil, and Other Antidepressants with Safe, Effective Alternatives*, published in 2000, included chapters on antidepressant withdrawal reactions and antidepressant-induced suicide and violence.[33] While *Prozac Backlash* called attention to these serious antidepressant side effects, no one could have predicted how large an international health problem they would become in just a few years. Physicians are increasingly concerned about malpractice lawsuits stemming from poorly managed withdrawal reactions and antidepressant-induced suicidality. Lawsuits, including class actions, involving thousands of patients who have suffered severe antidepressant withdrawal reactions, have been filed against the pharmaceutical industry so far in twenty-seven of fifty states. While my earlier book raised the withdrawal issue, which in 2000 was just coming to the attention of doctors and the public, this book provides the step-by-step solution. Since antidepressant-induced suicidality has become such a serious public health concern, a whole chapter is devoted to this topic and applies to any change in the dose, up or down.

As a clinical instructor in psychiatry at Harvard Medical School, a psychiatrist at the Harvard University Health Services, and a private practitioner in Harvard Square, I prescribe antidepressants regularly and have had countless patients report their benefits. At the same time, I have raised concerns that antidepressants are overprescribed for the stresses of everyday life and that patients are not adequately warned of their risks, including withdrawal reactions, suicide, and violence. Through my work with patients, physicians, and the media, I became aware of the need for a step-by-step guide to tapering antidepressants. Many patients and physicians have difficulty getting accurate information on antidepressant withdrawal reactions. This book is based on extensive experience tapering patients off antidepressants, input from colleagues with similar experience, and an exhaustive review of the medical literature on the subject. I also cite some pharmaceutical company documents that have become public record as a result of lawsuits.

This book presents a 5-Step Antidepressant Tapering Program developed over the years as I worked with many patients weaning off the drugs. The same guidelines apply when patients decrease the dose of their antidepressant in midtreatment. It is intended for anyone interested in or affected by antidepressant withdrawal and dependence:

- Patients on antidepressants who are ready to go off the drugs
- Patients who are considering going on antidepressants and are looking for more information on their potential side effects before making a decision
- Family doctors who are often unfamiliar with how to carefully taper the drugs
- Pediatricians who prescribe antidepressants to children and adolescents
- Psychiatrists
- Psychiatric nurses (who now do much of the prescribing in the mental health departments of HMOs)

- Psychotherapists, including social workers and psychologists, supporting patients through antidepressant withdrawal reactions
- Emergency room doctors and nurses who are frequently the first to see patients in the throes of antidepressant withdrawal
- Pharmacists whom patients often turn to with questions about their medications
- Family and friends who need support and accurate information because they often bear the brunt when patients in withdrawal become quite ill, irritable, or impulsive and behave in baffling, out-of-character ways

This book is intended to be helpful to doctors and patients alike. For this reason, I shift back and forth quite readily between addressing doctors and patients. In every instance, it is clear who is being addressed. Technical jargon has been minimized in order to provide a practical, straightforward approach to weaning patients off antidepressants. In some instances, I repeat important concepts and terms for readers who lack medical training. I trust readers with more medical knowledge will be understanding of my effort to make the information as accessible to as many people as possible. For those interested in more technical information, notes (which can be found at the back of the book) cite the extensive published medical reports and scientific research on antidepressant withdrawal and dependence.

Tapering antidepressants by following the guidelines of the 5-Step Antidepressant Tapering Program reduces both the incidence and severity of withdrawal reactions. Research has shown that when patients stop antidepressants cold turkey they can have high rates of withdrawal reactions, which vary depending on the particular drug. In studies involving hundreds of patients, 66 percent of patients stopping Paxil, 60 percent of patients stopping Zoloft, and 78 percent of patients stopping Effexor have withdrawal reactions.[34] Unfortunately, most doctors and patients have not been adequately informed about the problem of antidepressant withdrawal reactions. Under these circumstances, not surprisingly patients suffer high rates of withdrawal symptoms, including severe reactions. However, following the guidelines of the tapering program, in my experience most patients have no withdrawal reaction at all or mild withdrawal reactions that they tolerate comfortably.

The concern with withdrawal reactions should not overshadow the beneficial effects many patients report with antidepressants. Medications are not "bad" because they cause withdrawal symptoms when stopped too quickly. Other important classes of medications that can cause withdrawal reactions are blood pressure medications and anticonvulsants. With these drugs, doctors are familiar with how to taper them. While the magnitude of the problem of withdrawal and dependence with today's antidepressants has caught doctors and patients largely by surprise and is one the pharmaceutical industry has sought to minimize or deny, it is a problem that has to be confronted honestly and directly. The good news is that with proper information, doctors and patients can almost always safely and effectively overcome antidepressant withdrawal and dependence. Indeed, once patients are ready to go off antidepressants, tapering them over time provides a wonderful opportunity for collaboration, joint decision making, and strengthening the doctor-patient relationship that is at the heart of good medicine.

1

Antidepressant Withdrawal and Dependence

Defining the Problem

How Antidepressant Withdrawal Can Masquerade as Your Original Psychiatric Condition

"What do you mean I'm in Zoloft withdrawal?" Diana protested. "I went down on my Zoloft dose three days ago and now I'm depressed, I cry so easily, I'm anxious, I can't sleep . . . the same symptoms I went on Zoloft for six years ago. That's just my depression and anxiety coming back, isn't it?"

"Not necessarily," I responded. "They're also symptoms of antidepressant withdrawal."

"Antidepressant withdrawal! I didn't know such a thing existed. My previous doctor never said I could go into withdrawal if I tried to stop my antidepressant." Many doctors have not been taught that the kind of symptoms Diana was experiencing shortly after lowering the dose of her antidepressant are drug-induced withdrawal phenomena. Doctors and patients who are unaware of antidepressant withdrawal can mistake the symptoms for a return of the patient's original psychiatric condition, leading to years of additional unnecessary treatment. Studies have shown that as many as 78 percent of patients have withdrawal reactions when they stop their antidepressants, depending on the particular drug.[1]

Diana was a forty-seven-year-old newly named professor at Harvard who had recently moved with her husband and two teenage sons from Ann Arbor, Michigan for her new position. When Diana's move to Cambridge went smoothly, she wanted to try going off Zoloft as part of making a "fresh start" in life. Her new family doctor suggested reducing her dose from 150 to 100 milligrams a day. Three days later, she was in his office in a panic because she thought she was depressed and anxious again. The family doctor referred Diana to me because of my interest in antidepressant withdrawal.

"This happened to me twice back in Michigan," said Diana, still grappling with the idea that her symptoms were antidepressant withdrawal. "Once I tried to go off Zoloft and the other time I went on vacation and forgot to pack it."

"And you became symptomatic?"

"Both times I got exactly the same symptoms: I couldn't sleep. I was a mess, crying all the time. I felt depressed and anxious. Was that antidepressant withdrawal, too?"

"Did the symptoms start within days of changing your dose, like they did this time?"

Diana nodded. "Like clockwork, on day three."

"Then you were very likely in withdrawal, not a depressive relapse."

"I guess my doctor in Michigan didn't know about withdrawal. Instead, he confirmed my worst fear: That I was a hopeless case because I so quickly became depressed and anxious again without the drug."

Antidepressant withdrawal symptoms typically appear suddenly within days to weeks of lowering the dose, as in Diana's case. By contrast, when relapse occurs—a return of the patient's original psychiatric condition—it typically takes one to two months or more to slowly develop.[2] In addition, Diana had one of the most telltale medical symptoms of withdrawal: She was dizzy. Diana felt like "water was sloshing around" in her head and "the room was spinning." The characteristic dizziness was another important clue that Diana was in withdrawal rather than having a depressive relapse. Like many patients, Diana had overlooked the dizziness—until I asked specifically—because she was in such a panic over her psychiatric withdrawal symptoms.

Diana originally went on Zoloft because she became depressed and anxious after her son Jason was struck by a car and needed a series of operations to repair broken bones in his pelvis and legs. For almost a year Diana lived not only with the stress of Jason's surgeries, but also with the uncertainty of whether or not he would ever walk normally again. Because of the strain, her family doctor prescribed 100 milligrams a day of Zoloft, which helped her get through that difficult period in her life.

Diana first tried to go off Zoloft after Jason had recovered from his surgeries, was walking again, and was "completely out of the woods." Diana wanted to stop the antidepressant because she was having significant side effects: She had gained forty pounds and had lost all interest in sex with her husband to the point of aversion toward him. Both the weight gain and sexual dysfunction were deeply distressing to her. With Jason's difficulties behind her, she was confident she could do without the drug.

To Diana's dismay, within days of stopping Zoloft she became anxious, tearful, and unable to sleep. Because her doctor in Michigan mistook antidepressant withdrawal for a depressive relapse, he not only put her back on the drug, he increased Diana's dose to 150 milligrams a day.

A few months later, Diana forgot to pack her Zoloft when she went out of town for a long weekend with her husband. Again, she became tearful, irritable, and jittery. By the time she got home she was "desperate" for Zoloft. Her symptoms disappeared within hours of taking the drug. At that point, Diana mistakenly concluded her psychiatric condition was far worse than it actually was.

"I've been on Zoloft for six years," said Diana. "After the first two years, I tried to go off the Zoloft and was forced back on it because of withdrawal. Does that mean that for four of the six years I've been taking Zoloft . . . ," I could almost see the gears turning in Diana's head as she made the calculation, "I've been using it to medicate withdrawal instead of to treat my original depression and anxiety?"

"It seems so." Of course, had Diana successfully tapered off the Zoloft, she might have had a depressive relapse months later. But I explained why I thought this highly unlikely: "Your stress was due to the crisis caused by Jason's accident. It sounds like you no longer needed the Zoloft once the crisis was over, once Jason was okay and you were no longer worried about him. When you tried to stop the Zoloft and had to go back on it because of withdrawal symptoms you were clearly taking the medication to suppress uncomfortable withdrawal, not to treat your original depression and anxiety. If we taper you off Zoloft and you do fine without it—you don't become depressed or anxious again—then your last four years on the drug probably were unnecessary. It's a tragedy that pharmaceutical companies haven't better educated doctors and the public about antidepressant withdrawal so that you didn't have to go through those four years."

Diana shook her head, stunned.

When patients have to restart antidepressants, put the dose back up, or taper off them more slowly because of withdrawal, they are no longer taking the drugs for therapeutic reasons to treat their psychiatric conditions. Instead, they are using the drugs to suppress intolerable withdrawal reactions. The technical, medical term for this is "dependence" because the patients cannot do without the drugs until they manage to wean off them.[3] Diana was right: She had been dependent on Zoloft for four of the six years she was on it, when she no longer needed it and was instead taking the drug to suppress withdrawal.

Diana and I had no choice but to put her dose back up to 150 milligrams a day because her withdrawal symptoms became so severe. Once she was back on the drug, her withdrawal symptoms cleared within twenty-four hours. Diana took weeks to recover from the episode of withdrawal and the shock of having been on the drug needlessly for years. Once she had fully recovered, we tapered her much more slowly off Zoloft over the course of four months. We followed the 5-Step Antidepressant Tapering Program detailed in subsequent chapters of this guide for doctors and patients. Diana has been off Zoloft for three years and has not had any return of depression or anxiety, confirming that she had no longer needed the drug once the crisis with her son was resolved.

Off Zoloft, Diana lost the forty pounds she had gained and revived her sex life with her husband. In retrospect Diana says: "I'm still grateful for the help Zoloft gave me that first year when I was a wreck over Jason. But I'm angry that my doctor didn't know about withdrawal so I could have gotten off the drug once I no longer needed it. The weight gain and sexual problems were making me miserable. I switched doctors only because I moved. If I hadn't, I might have stayed on Zoloft for the rest of my life."

The Antidepressant Catch-22

Countless patients are caught in the antidepressant catch-22 that Diana was in: restarting antidepressants or putting the dose back up thinking they are treating depression when, in fact, they have become dependent on the drugs to suppress withdrawal reactions. We do not know exactly how many people are caught in this dilemma, because it has not been studied systematically. Studies have shown that 30 to 60 percent of patients forget to take their antidepressants for a few days or more.[4] If a third of these patients, a conservative estimate, experience withdrawal symptoms that they mistake for relapse of their original psychiatric conditions, then they are in the position Diana was in. With 20 million people on the drugs, one can reasonably estimate that millions of people may be trapped in this dilemma.[5]

Still other patients become caught in the antidepressant catch-22 because they forget to take their medication for a few days, call their doctors because they are feeling depressed and anxious, and do not think to even mention missing doses of their antidepressant. They report: "I'm feeling worse despite being on an antidepressant." Their doctors, not attuned to the withdrawal phenomena, jump to the conclusion: "You need to go up on the dose."

Being caught in the antidepressant catch-22 needlessly exposes patients—often for years—to the side effects and long-term risks of antidepressants. In many instances, not only is the drug restarted, the dose is increased and additional drugs—additional antidepressants, lithium, anticonvulsants, thyroid hormone, Ritalin, and other stimulants—are added to "treat" withdrawal that has been mistaken for a depressive relapse. In the process, patients get the false impression that their psychiatric conditions and prognoses are far worse than they actually are. For patients trapped in this dilemma, the result is profound human suffering with broad social ramifications.[6] Lastly, treating patients needlessly with antidepressants, while a boon for the pharmaceutical industry, is a costly burden on the financially strapped health care system.

Some patients and their doctors do accurately diagnose antidepressant withdrawal. But when the patients are forced to restart the drugs or to go back up on the dose, the doctors do not know what to do next. Ed is a forty-four-year-old auto mechanic whose doctor tried to "taper" him off of 40 milligrams a day of Paxil in just three weeks. Ed ended up with severe nausea, vomiting, dizziness, imbalance, and electric shock–like "zaps" in his brain. Ed's withdrawal symptoms were so debilitating that he became bedridden and lost two days of work before his doctor finally put his Paxil dose back up. The symptoms began to clear within hours of his restarting the drug. Once Ed was feeling better, his doctor suggested "tapering" Paxil by alternating days on and days off the drug. Ed began alternating taking 40 milligrams of Paxil one day and not the next. This regimen produced a "roller coaster" of on-again off-again withdrawal symptoms that once again forced Ed to go on 40 milligrams a day. In fact, alternating days on and days off is no way to taper an antidepressant like Paxil but, like many family doctors, Ed's family doctor was unaware. Finally, Ed's doctor acknowledged: "I don't know what to do. I tried tapering you a couple of different ways and it hasn't worked." Ed's doctor eventually referred him to me. Rather than trying to do it in three weeks, we successfully tapered Ed off the Paxil over the course of three months. Ed has been off Paxil for four years and has not suffered a relapse into depression.

The fact that antidepressant withdrawal can mimic a patient's original psychiatric condition is a cruel irony that requires doctors and patients to be well informed and vigilant about distinguishing antidepressant withdrawal from depressive relapse.[7] Yet a 1997 study published in the *Journal of Clinical Psychiatry* found that 70 percent of family doctors are not aware of antidepressant withdrawal, even though they write the vast majority of prescriptions for antidepressants.[8] Since then, the situation has improved some but not nearly enough. Many family doctors do not know how severe antidepressant withdrawal can be and how slowly some patients need to taper off the drugs.

Detailed studies and scores of reports of antidepressant withdrawal have been published in medical journals. One large-scale, systematic study conducted at Harvard Medical School in 1998 found that 66 percent of patients taking Paxil and 60 percent of patients taking Zoloft developed withdrawal reactions if they stopped their drug or forgot to take it for just a few days.[9] In another study of Paxil conducted by the British equivalent of our FDA, 21 percent of Paxil withdrawal reactions were mild, 58 percent were moderately severe, and 21 percent were severe.[10] Of the patients who experienced Paxil withdrawal, 57 percent had to restart the drug because of moderately severe or severe withdrawal symptoms. When discussing antidepressant withdrawal and dependence, Paxil is often used as the reference drug because it is the antidepressant most commonly associated with withdrawal reactions.[11] In another study, 40 percent of patients in antidepressant withdrawal had incapacitating withdrawal symptoms that kept them out of work, 25 percent sought urgent medical attention, and 50 percent called their doctors for reassurance.[12] These sobering statistics testify to the magnitude of the problem. Unfortunately, many of the studies of antidepressant withdrawal and dependence have been published in obscure academic journals and are not well known, even among doctors.

Experts divide antidepressant withdrawal symptoms into two main categories: psychiatric symptoms and medical symptoms.[13] The psychiatric symptoms of antidepressant withdrawal include depressed mood, low energy, crying uncontrollably, anxiety, insomnia, irritability, agitation, impulsivity, hallucinations, or suicidal and violent urges. In March 2004, the FDA warned that antidepressant withdrawal reactions may make patients suicidal.[14] Even before the FDA warning, there were reports published in medical journals of patients having antidepressant withdrawal reactions who became homicidal, had suicidal thoughts, and made suicide attempts.[15] The medical symptoms of antidepressant withdrawal include disabling dizziness, imbalance, nausea, vomiting, flu-like aches and pains, sweating, headaches, tremors, burning sensations, or electric shock–like "zaps" in the brain. Since the symptoms of antidepressant withdrawal can include suicidal urges, withdrawal can be a life-threatening medical emergency.

Antidepressant withdrawal correlates with how quickly the drugs are excreted from the body—how quickly they "wash out"—once patients stop taking them.[16] Even after patients no longer need antidepressants to treat their original psychiatric conditions, their brain cells still need time to readjust to stopping the drugs. Stopping antidepressants abruptly or lowering the dose precipitously does not give brain cells adequate time to readjust.[17] The resulting stress on the brain cells causes antidepressant withdrawal symptoms. Even when patients experience few or no withdrawal symptoms, their brain cells are still adjusting to living with less of the drug. So far, research has only just begun to look at this complex physiological process; we do not yet fully understand the subtleties of how the nervous system readjusts to declining levels of antidepressants. For example, antidepressants can cause abnormal eye movements during sleep that persist for over a year *after* an antidepressant is stopped.[18] If some antidepressant effects can persist that long after the drugs are stopped, giving the nervous system adequate time to readjust after each dosage reduction may be an essential element in tapering off the drugs safely and effectively.

Carefully tapering antidepressants over a reasonable period of time may also provide protection against depressive relapse at a later date. Studies have shown that in the early months after patients stop psychiatric drugs abruptly, they are at increased risk of relapse, or recurrence, of their original psychiatric condition, in excess of the natural course of the illness if it had gone untreated.[19] The excess risk is thought to be due to the negative effects on brain cells caused by stopping the drugs abruptly.

Tapering slowly off antidepressants reduces the negative effects on brain cells. In my experience, patients who follow the guidelines of the 5-Step Antidepressant Tapering Program have a low incidence of depressive relapse after going off the drugs.

The tremendous unpredictability of antidepressant withdrawal reactions from one person to the next is part of what makes tapering antidepressants so difficult. While one patient may be able to taper off of 20 milligrams a day of Paxil in six weeks, the next patient on the same dose may take six months to taper off the drug. If a patient experiences mild withdrawal reactions, he may be able to reduce the dose in 10-milligram increments, from 20 to 10 to 0 milligrams a day in less than two months. But if a patient experiences severe withdrawal reactions, he may be able to reduce the dose only in small, 2.5-milligram increments, from 20 to 17.5 to 15 and so on over the course of many months. This extraordinarily wide variation requires doctors to customize the size of dosage reductions and the time frame of the taper for each patient. This is one of the more difficult aspects of tapering antidepressants and one of the reasons why the subject warrants a book such as this.

Until now, detailed guidelines for doctors and patients on how to taper antidepressants have been lacking. The few guidelines that do exist are little known and not flexible or detailed enough. For example, the *Drug and Therapeutics Bulletin* recommends fixed antidepressant dosage reductions of 25 percent every four to six weeks.[20] But in reality the amount by which the dose can be reduced varies widely from one patient to the next. If a patient has mild antidepressant withdrawal reactions, she may be able to reduce the dose by 50 percent. But if a patient has severe antidepressant withdrawal reactions, she may be able to reduce the dose only by 10 percent or less. Other guidelines recommend specific time frames. One well-known textbook of psychiatry recommends tapering over the course of just one to two weeks.[21] But two weeks is an unrealistically short time.

One general rule of thumb sometimes used to taper drugs that cause withdrawal is the "ten percent rule": reducing the dose by 10 percent every seven to ten days. But why resign yourself to such a slow taper lasting months if, in fact, you are one of the fortunate ones who could make a much larger, 50 percent reduction and be off your antidepressant in less than two months? The sensible way to wean antidepressants is a highly flexible program, like the 5-Step Antidepressant Tapering Program detailed in this book, which provides recommended tapering schedules for all of the antidepressants currently on the market together with guidelines for carefully monitoring the patient's withdrawal symptoms and slowing the taper down, making smaller reductions, if necessary.

Why do some people experience more severe antidepressant withdrawal and dependence than others? Antidepressants wash out of the body by being inactivated in the liver and then being excreted in the urine. We now know that people vary widely in how quickly or slowly their livers metabolize, or inactivate, antidepressants. Recent research has focused on the enzymes in the liver that metabolize antidepressants. Some people with robust enzymes are "fast metabolizers" of antidepressants, while others with sluggish enzymes are "slow metabolizers." Fast metabolizers may be more prone to antidepressant withdrawal because the drugs wash out more quickly, leaving brain cells inadequate time to adjust.[22] Other factors may play a role as well: Some patients' brain cells may be more sensitive than others to falling levels of antidepressants.[23]

Antidepressants should always be tapered following appropriate protocols and under careful medical supervision.[24] Due to the growing problem of antidepressant withdrawal and dependence, some pharmaceutical companies have added warnings to their official information on antidepressants. Unfortunately, the warnings are often very general, written in fine print, and fall short in alerting doctors and patients to the problem and providing them with guidelines for coping with it. For example, GlaxoSmithKline now cautions that Paxil should be discontinued by "a gradual reduction in the dose rather than abrupt cessation."[25] But the "guidelines" the company provides for tapering the drug simply state: "If intolerable symptoms occur following a decrease in the dose or upon discontinuation of treatment, then *resuming the previously prescribed dose may be considered.* Subsequently, the physician may continue decreasing the dose *but at a more gradual rate* [emphasis added]." Obviously such a vague statement offers little in the way of helping doctors and patients decide how much to reduce the dose and in what time frame.

The 5-Step Antidepressant Tapering Program

The good news is that patients can almost always wean off antidepressants comfortably and safely by carefully tapering them.[26] The five-step program presented here provides step-by-step guidelines for gradually lowering the dose of antidepressants and for customizing the time frame and size of dosage reductions for each individual patient. Subsequent chapters describe in detail:

- How to recognize and monitor antidepressant withdrawal symptoms
- How to distinguish the psychiatric symptoms of withdrawal from depressive relapse
- How to distinguish the medical symptoms of withdrawal from other medical conditions
- How to determine the optional size dosage reduction for you
- How long to wait between dosage reductions
- How to establish a routine of comfortable size dosage reductions at reasonable time intervals
- How to adjust the tapering schedule to proceed more quickly or slowly depending on the severity of your withdrawal symptoms

Carefully tapering antidepressants reduces both the incidence and severity of withdrawal symptoms. How long the taper requires depends on the particular antidepressant you are taking, how long you have been on the drug, how high your dose is at the start of the taper, and your sensitivity to withdrawal symptoms. The goal of tapering is to reduce your discomfort and increase your safety while weaning off an antidepressant. Most patients are able to complete the 5-Step Antidepressant Tapering Program in two to four months. Patients who experience mild withdrawal reactions may be able to complete the program in less than two months. Other patients who experience severe withdrawal reactions may take four to six months.

When patients stop antidepressants cold turkey they can have high rates of withdrawal reactions, depending on the particular drug: 66 percent of patients stopping Paxil, 60 percent of patients stopping Zoloft, and 78 percent of patients stopping Effexor have withdrawal reactions.[27] Since most doctors and patients have not been adequately informed about antidepressant withdrawal reactions, many patients suffer high rates of withdrawal reactions, including severe withdrawal. However, in my experience with patients following the guidelines of the 5-Step Antidepressant Tapering Program, most have no withdrawal reaction or mild withdrawal reactions that are comfortably tolerated.

In addition to preventing severe withdrawal reactions, tapering antidepressants also cushions people psychologically as they let go of drugs they have relied on, often for some time. Most patients, no matter how well they are doing, have some fear of "rocking the boat" by going off their antidepressant. Making measured reductions in the medication over reasonable periods of time reassures patients that nothing dramatic is happening as they gradually adjust to living without the medication.

Antidepressant withdrawal and dependence affect people of all ages, men and women, regardless of the diagnosis for which they were put on the drugs. Patients stopping antidepressants can have withdrawal reactions even if the drugs did not work—did not help their psychiatric condition—while they were on them.[28] Antidepressant withdrawal and dependence can occur in patients on very low doses, even doses below the minimum recommended by pharmaceutical companies.[29] There are published reports of patients who simply could not get off their antidepressants because their withdrawal reactions were so severe.[30] Some people describe tapering their antidepressant down to a low dose, like 2.5 milligrams a day of Paxil, but then being "stuck" there, unable to lower the dose further because of severe withdrawal reactions.[31] While withdrawal symptoms typically peak and disappear within two to three weeks, there are published reports of patients whose withdrawal symptoms lasted for months after they stopped antidepressants.[32] Young children appear to be more vulnerable to antidepressant withdrawal than adults.[33] Experts believe this is because their metabolism is faster. Newborns whose mothers were taking antidepressants during pregnancy can have withdrawal reactions shortly after birth.[34] Similarly, breastfeeding infants whose mothers abruptly stop antidepressants can have severe withdrawal reactions.[35]

Anyone who has been on an antidepressant for more than about a month can experience withdrawal symptoms and dependence if the drug is stopped abruptly.[36] Patients with severe withdrawal symptoms feel "held hostage" to the drugs because it can take months to painstakingly wean off them. Patients often have to cut their antidepressant pills into fragments—quarters, halves, even eighths—to get smaller and smaller doses with which to taper their drugs. No one can predict in advance which patients will have the most severe withdrawal reactions, so all patients need to cautiously taper off the drugs.

Withdrawal reactions can occur when patients:

• Decrease the dose in midtreatment or when tapering off antidepressants

- Stop antidepressants abruptly
- Accidentally forget or skip doses

Even when patients taper carefully, many still experience withdrawal symptoms, but the symptoms are less severe than if they stopped suddenly or lowered the dose too quickly. Some patients have to slow down the pace of a taper as they get to lower doses in order to remain comfortable. When patients decrease the dose of an antidepressant in midtreatment, they need to follow the same guidelines and precautions that they do when decreasing the dose to taper off the drug.

As seen in Table 1.1, most of today's popular antidepressants are members of a class known as selective serotonin reuptake inhibitors, or SSRIs, because they are promoted as increasing the brain chemical serotonin. The original member of the group, Prozac, became popular in the early 1990s.[37] The antidepressants in the group now include Prozac, Zoloft, Paxil, Celexa, Lexapro, and Luvox, all of which cause antidepressant withdrawal to varying degrees.[38] Three other antidepressants are closely related to the SSRIs: Effexor, Cymbalta, and Serzone are promoted as increasing the brain chemicals serotonin and noradrenalin, the form of adrenalin found in the brain.[39] Effexor, Cymbalta, and Serzone are therefore known as SNRIs, selective serotonin and noradrenalin reuptake inhibitors. Serzone has been linked to cases of liver failure and the

Table 1.1 CLASSES OF TODAY'S POPULAR ANTIDEPRESSANTS

Selective Serotonin Reuptake Inhibitors (SSRIs)	Paxil Zoloft Prozac Celexa Lexapro Luvox
Serotonin and Noradrenalin Reuptake Inhibitors (SNRIs)	Effexor Cymbalta Serzone
Other	Wellbutrin Remeron

brand name version of the drug was pulled from the market in the spring of 2004, although the generic version remains available.[40] Remeron boosts serotonin and noradrenalin, but by a different mechanism, the details of which are not important for our purposes.[41] Finally, Wellbutrin boosts still another brain chemical, called dopamine.[42] The FDA's March 2004 warning that antidepressant withdrawal reactions may make patients suicidal applies to all eleven of these antidepressants—Prozac, Zoloft, Paxil, Celexa, Lexapro, Luvox, Effexor, Cymbalta, Serzone, Remeron, and Wellbutrin. While these drugs are the focus of this book, Appendix 3 discusses tapering the older class of antidepressants, called tricyclic antidepressants (many of which are still in use today), and Appendix 4 discusses still another class of antidepressants, monoamine oxidase inhibitors (MAOIs).

Paxil, Effexor, and Wellbutrin also come in slow, or controlled, release forms called Paxil CR, Effexor XR, Wellbutrin SR, and Wellbutrin XL. Some doctors and patients mistakenly think that the slow release forms of antidepressants protect against withdrawal, but this is not the case.[43] They too need to be tapered carefully.

When patients switch from one SSRI or SNRI to another antidepressant in the same class, they may not experience withdrawal symptoms. The new antidepressant may protect against withdrawal from the old one because they are in the same class. However, this is not the case if one switches to an antidepressant in a different class.

When Prozac was introduced, doctors thought it rarely caused withdrawal and dependence. We now know withdrawal reactions are not rare with Prozac. Studies have shown withdrawal reactions occur in 14 percent of patients stopping Prozac.[44] Still, this is a much lower rate than with other antidepressants. Prozac causes fewer withdrawal reactions because when stopped, it gradually washes out of the body over the course of weeks, providing a slow, built-in taper. By contrast, other currently popular antidepressants wash out precipitously, over the course of hours and days, often leaving brain cells too little time to adjust. Antidepressant withdrawal and dependence have come to the attention of doctors and the public only since the introduction of the much shorter–acting drugs in the class. In fact, one reason doctors have been slow to recognize the severity of the problem is because of assumptions made early on based on Prozac.

In the decades before Prozac appeared in the 1990s, earlier classes of antidepressants were well known to cause withdrawal reactions when stopped abruptly.[45] In those "old days," psychiatrists routinely tapered patients off of antidepressants over the course of months. In many ways, this book is about rediscovering the lost art of tapering antidepressants. The book not only revives the skill but applies it specifically to today's antidepressants. This is especially important for family doctors, who now write the majority of antidepressant prescriptions. As it was chiefly psychiatrists, not family doctors, who prescribed the earlier agents, family doctors have little experience with the protocols used to taper patients off antidepressants. In the Afterword, we will look more closely at why the skill of tapering antidepressants was lost.

Among psychiatrists, only the "older generation" with experience prescribing antidepressants before the 1990s is familiar with tapering antidepressants. The generation that entered the field in the last fifteen years has little experience with the earlier classes of antidepressants and therefore with tapering the drugs. Finally, at the mental health services of HMOs, psychiatric nurses do much of the prescribing of antidepressants nowadays. This is a relatively recent trend. As a result, psychiatric nurses, too, have little experience tapering antidepressants. The net result is that the majority of clinicians prescribing antidepressants nowadays are not familiar with how to taper the drugs when patients no longer need them.

When some people hear tapering off antidepressants can take months, they are astonished: "It takes only weeks, not months, to be detoxed off alcohol and other street drugs. How can it take longer to get off antidepressants?" The difference is that when people enter alcohol detox and rehabilitation programs, they go into the hospital or they enter intensive day treatment programs. They interrupt their daily lives, taking time off from work or school. Often, they are extremely uncomfortable and at risk for delirium tremens and seizures. Instead, we are talking about people carefully tapering off antidepressants while continuing to go about their everyday lives. The point of tapering antidepressants carefully is so that people remain relatively comfortable and can continue to function as close to normally as possible.

Patients who have good experiences with antidepressants and have not yet tried to go off them, or who went off them with mild withdrawal symptoms, are sometimes surprised by the severe withdrawal reactions other patients experience. "It doesn't sound like the same drug I was taking," say some patients. But this is true of many prescription drugs: some people have few side effects while others have horrendous side effects. This is a reality that should not negate either the positive stories some people recount or the terrible stories others have to tell. The risk-benefit ratio of antidepressants—their side effects versus therapeutic effects— also varies considerably for different patients. Patients whose treatment brought them back from the brink of suicidal depressions may be a lot more accepting of having to taper painstakingly slowly off antidepressants than patients who were prescribed the drugs for mild conditions that might have been treated without medication.

The decision to taper off antidepressants requires a careful clinical evaluation and needs to be made jointly by patients and doctors, as discussed in Chapter 7. Psychiatrists generally recommend that when antidepressants work for patients, they should remain on them for a minimum of six months before trying to go off.[46] Many patients are on antidepressants longer. If your doctor knows little about antidepressant withdrawal and dependence, encourage him or her to learn more about it with you. If your doctor is not prepared to discuss the possibility of reducing the dose of your antidepressant, you can always seek a second opinion.

The antidepressant catch-22—patients who are needlessly dependent on antidepressants and do not realize it—is a hidden national health care crisis within the larger problem of antidepressant withdrawal and dependence. All patients on antidepressants for more than a year should have a thorough clinical evaluation to determine if they are trapped in this catch-22. The goal of an evaluation is to establish whether the patient and her doctor have ever mistaken withdrawal symptoms for a relapse of the original psychiatric condition and restarted the drug, increased the dose, or added additional antidepressants to suppress withdrawal symptoms. A patient caught in the antidepressant catch-22 should be evaluated to see if it would be an appropriate time to enter a tapering program to try going off the drug.

People who want to try going off today's antidepressants are usually either feeling better and believe they no longer need the drugs, or are having significant side effects. Substantial weight gain is one of the most common problems prompting patients to stop their antidepressants.[47] Sexual side effects—ranging from mild loss of libido to severe sexual dysfunction—occur in as many as 60 percent or more of patients, depending on the particular drug.[48] When patients first go on antidepressants, they often feel stimulated or "caffeinated." But with time, many people develop a "bone weary" fatigue that leaves them feeling sluggish.[49] Antidepressants stop working in about a third of patients.[50]

Even people who are not having significant side effects may be concerned about the risks of taking antidepressants indefinitely. In April 2003, *Glamour* magazine ran an article entitled "Addicted to Antidepressants?"[51] The article featured people who had experienced debilitating antidepressant withdrawal, including twenty-nine-year-old Adrienne Bransky of Chicago. Although grateful that Paxil had brought her back from the brink of a suicidal depression, Bransky spoke for many patients when she reflected: "Most people don't want to rely on antidepressants all their lives. We all hold out the hope that we won't have to take these pills forever. That's why pharmaceutical companies need to be more forthright and responsible and need to put more money into educating doctors about the risks of withdrawal. Maybe then you'll have fewer patients going through the [withdrawal] hell I went through." The purpose of this book is to spare patients the kind of "withdrawal hell" Bransky and others have gone through.

2

Resolving the Controversy over "Addiction" to Antidepressants
The BBC Exposé

Steven the Self-Proclaimed "Paxil Junkie"

"How long ago did you call Dr. Glenmullen?" Steven asked his wife, Anne, impatiently.

"Fifteen minutes."

"Can you call him again?"

"Steven, I can't keep calling him every fifteen minutes. It's Saturday night. He's probably not home."

"I've got to have some Paxil!" Steven insisted, desperately. In severe Paxil withdrawal, Steven had not been able to leave his apartment all day because of debilitating dizziness and headaches. Steven was so dizzy he felt "trapped" on his living room couch, unable to get up even to walk around the room. His head felt like water was sloshing around inside it; just turning it to talk to Anne made the dizziness worse. Steven's pounding head felt like it had been "split open with an axe." He had taken several doses of Tylenol with codeine, but the potent painkiller had not remedied the headaches. Steven's body was wracked with severe aches and pains in his joints. He felt sapped of all energy.

When Anne sat down beside Steven and tenderly put her arm around him, he irritably brushed her off. "What's come over you?" asked Anne, startled.

"I don't feel like being touched, I feel so awful." A gentle giant by nature, Steven's irritability was out of character and another symptom of Paxil withdrawal.

Moving further away on the couch to give Steven more space, Anne opened a magazine. A few minutes later, Steven snapped: "Will you please leave?"

"Why?"

"Your reading."

"What's wrong with my reading?"

"I can't stand the noise of the pages turning."

"The noise?"

"Every time you turn a page, the noise reverberates in my head. Every page feels like someone dropped a brick on my head."

"Because of your headache?" Anne tried to comprehend what Steven was experiencing.

"Yes!"

Realizing how wretched Steven felt, Anne went into the couple's bedroom and tried to reach me again. She left another message saying how desperately Steven was in need of Paxil. Returning to the living room, she and Steven began to discuss alternatives, other ways they might get ahold of the drug. Anne telephoned the pharmacy wondering if the pharmacist could give her just a few pills for Steven. The pharmacist said no, she could not dispense the antidepressant without a prescription, and suggested going to the emergency room of the Mount Auburn Hospital, near where the couple lived in Cambridge. Steven hated the thought of leaving the house because he felt so sick. As the couple debated whether or not to go to the emergency room, I retrieved Anne's messages and returned her call.

"We're so relieved to hear from you," Anne declared, handing the phone to Steven.

"You warned me about withdrawal," said Steven with a mixture of exasperation over his situation and relief to hear from me, "but I never would have believed it could be this bad, that I could feel this desperate for a drug."

Steven had stopped 20 milligrams a day of Paxil just a few days earlier, on Wednesday. On Friday, he first noticed feeling dizzy while walking along a crowded street in Harvard Square. The dizziness was so disorienting that Steven feared he might fall into the oncoming crowd. On Friday evening, he developed severe aches and pains in his muscles and joints. Initially, he thought he had the flu, but when he awoke on Saturday morning with the pounding headache he realized he was in Paxil withdrawal. Steven felt so drained of energy that he had to cancel his Saturday morning workout at the gym. "I never cancel my workout," said Steven. "I'm religious about it. I have to be at death's door to cancel." Not wanting to bother me on a Saturday, Steven tried valiantly to "tough it out." But as the day went on, he felt worse and worse. By the evening he finally "succumbed to wanting Paxil" and "begged" Anne to telephone me.

Just a few months earlier, Steven had stopped smoking cigarettes cold turkey. He had been a heavy, one-to-two-pack-a-day smoker for nineteen years. He began exercising regularly at the gym at the same time that he gave up smoking as part of adopting a healthier lifestyle. Steven had been able to "tough out" giving up cigarettes, despite cigarette cravings, irritability, and feeling physically ill. Given his willpower in the face of nicotine withdrawal, Steven assumed he would have no trouble going off Paxil even if he did experience withdrawal. But, said Steven: "I couldn't do the same—stop cold turkey—with Paxil. It's humiliating to crave a drug so badly that you ask your wife to call a pharmacy to beg for it. . . . All day I've been completely preoccupied with getting Paxil. That's all I've been able to think about. I'm sorry for calling you on the weekend but there's no way I could have made it until Monday."

I reassured Steven that it was fine to call me under the circumstances and telephoned the pharmacy with a prescription for him. Anne went straightaway to pick it up. Within three hours of taking 20 milligrams of Paxil, all of Steven's withdrawal symptoms had disappeared except the headache, which, however, was dramatically improved. When he awoke on Sunday morning, the headache, too, was gone and Steven felt back to normal. Indeed, he was able to work out at the gym, which had been "inconceivable" the previous day when he was in severe withdrawal.

Anne accompanied Steven to his appointment with me on the following Tuesday. "Saturday was scary," said Anne, still shaken up by Steven's experience with Paxil withdrawal. "What if we hadn't been able to reach you? What if you were away for the weekend?" In fact, I **had** suggested to Steven that he slowly taper the Paxil. When he did not think that would be necessary, I offered to give him a prescription for the medication just in case, but he declined. In retrospect, Steven was overconfident of his ability to tough out any Paxil withdrawal he experienced because of his success in stopping smoking cigarettes.

"I was amazed by how quickly the withdrawal went away once I took just one Paxil," said Steven. "I had no real doubt, but that certainly confirmed I was in withdrawal."

"Did you try to treat the headaches with Tylenol with codeine?" I asked, recalling that Steven had said something to this effect when I spoke with him by phone on Saturday.

"Yes. It's called Tylenol 3."

"Codeine's a narcotic so it's very strong."

"That's how bad the headache was! The Tylenol 3 didn't touch it."

"Do you get bad headaches from time to time? Is that why you had the Tylenol 3?"

"No. I never get headaches. I had a few of the Tylenol 3 left over from when my wisdom teeth were pulled six months ago."

Both Steven and Anne are teachers from California who came to Harvard to get master's degrees in the School of Education. A psychiatrist in San Francisco originally started Steven on Paxil for depression. When he arrived in Cambridge, Steven came to see me for psychotherapy and renewals of his Paxil prescription. He decided to go off the Paxil because he and Anne wanted to begin trying to get pregnant. Paxil had "killed" Steven's sex drive and his ability to maintain an erection. At the time of that first attempt to go off Paxil, Steven had not been depressed for over a year.

Sobered by his terrible experience of antidepressant withdrawal, Steven was more determined than ever to go off Paxil. He was on the medication another five months before a painstakingly slow taper allowed him to wean off. Each time he stepped down his Paxil dose, he again experienced withdrawal symptoms, although not as severe as when he had tried to stop cold turkey. Each time he fell ill with headaches, dizziness, flu-like aches and pains, malaise, and irritability. He used Tylenol to blunt the headaches and toughed out the withdrawal symptoms for one to two weeks with each dosage reduction.

Two months into the taper, one night Steven and Anne were watching television when they saw an advertisement for Paxil. The ad featured a series of tense, anxious people gesticulating, fretting, shaking their heads, and rubbing their temples. One woman said she could not participate in life because she was so "bogged down with worry." Another said her anxiety was "like a tape in my head that just goes over and over and over." One man hung his head in defeat because he could not relax at work or at home. Then suddenly, after going on Paxil, the same people were flashing shiny, happy smiles. One woman kissed her son, tossed him in the air, and hoisted him up on her shoulders. Another decorated a cake with her daughter. The man who couldn't relax at work or at home now polished his vintage car with blissful satisfaction. The line in the Hallmark card–like ad that most enraged Steven was the explicit statement "Paxil is non–habit forming."

"How can they get away with that?" Steven railed at our next session. "I'm sitting there unable to get off Paxil for months watching them advertise it as non–habit forming? Sure my life is waiting for me . . . when I get off the drug. Until then, Anne and I can't move forward with trying to get pregnant. How can they make such false claims? I'm living proof Paxil is addicting. I'm hooked on Paxil. I'm a Paxil junkie!"

"You're not actually addicted to Paxil, even though you can't get off it," I gently explained to Steven.

"What am I, then?"

"You're dependent on it."

"Dependent. Hooked. Addicted. What's the difference?"

"You're dependent, because stopping the drug abruptly would cause you to have a debilitating withdrawal reaction, like you did the first weekend you tried to stop the Paxil."

"How's that different from being addicted?" asked Steven, confused.

"To be addicted you have to have cravings for a drug."

"I craved Paxil the weekend I tried to stop cold turkey. I was begging Anne to call you and the pharmacy, I craved it so bad."

The pharmaceutical industry has drummed into doctors and patients the idea that today's best-selling antidepressants are not addicting, according to the technical, medical definition of the term. Yet Steven had just refuted one of the grounds on which this claim is made. Reciting yet another tenet of the definition, I said, "When people are addicted to drugs, they use escalating doses."

"One of my best friends was on 20 milligrams a day of Paxil and it wore off. He went up to 40 milligrams and it wore off. He had to go up to 60 milligrams a day. He's worried about what he'll do if the 60 milligrams a day wears off, because that's the legal limit."

Again, Steven was right. Patients do develop tolerance to antidepressants and need higher doses. Indeed, one study done at Harvard Medical School found that Prozac wore off within a year in one-third of patients.[1]

Grasping at the last straw of the technical, medical definition of addiction, I argued, "When people are addicted to a drug, they use it to get high."

"I hear stories at the high school where I teach of students getting high on antidepressants like Paxil and Wellbutrin. They crush antidepressants and snort them like they snort cocaine."

This, too, is true, I realized as Steven spoke. One also hears these stories about students on college campuses.[2] In recent years, I have chaired town meeting–style forums on college campuses to discuss the high percentage of college students taking antidepressants. Invariably, a student or faculty member raises the topic of students abusing antidepressants in just the way Steven described. Until recently, antidepressant abuse was relatively uncommon, because antidepressants were still patented and actually more expensive than street drugs like cocaine. But, as the drugs' patents expire and they become cheaper, abuse may become more common. Indeed, the cover article "Generation Rx: Pop, Snort, Parachute" in the October 4, 2004 issue of *New York* magazine described New York teenagers abusing prescription drugs, including antidepressants.[3] The author interviewed more than fifty teenagers, many of whom stole the drugs from their parents' medicine cabinets. The "pills are more addictive than anyone realizes," the teens insisted.

Many patients "chip" their antidepressants in a milder form of abuse of the drugs.[4] "Chipping" is taking extra, unprescribed doses of antidepressants. Patients most often take extra doses in the late afternoon or evening to give them more energy and improve their concentration to get through difficult or boring stretches of work. The term "chipping" originally referred to taking extra shavings ("chips") of the crystalline form of an illegal street drug.

In subsequent meetings Steven continued to describe himself as "addicted" to Paxil, as do many patients who have difficulty stopping antidepressants. After a number of similar discussions with other patients I began to realize that, even according to the technical, medical definition, antidepressants can be "addicting." That is, patients can crave them when in withdrawal, can use escalating doses, and in some instances can even abuse them to get high. Still more importantly, the technical, medical definition is not what matters when it comes to advertising and marketing directed at patients. What matters is the plain-English definition of addiction when speaking to patients. The *Oxford English Dictionary* states that addiction is "having a compulsion to take a drug, the stopping of which produces withdrawal symptoms."[5] Withdrawal symptoms are precisely what afflict countless patients who try to stop antidepressants.[6]

Over the past decade, pharmaceutical companies and psychiatrists who are strong drug proponents have adamantly denied that antidepressants are addicting or habit forming. As antidepressant withdrawal began to come to the attention of doctors and patients in the mid-1990s, Eli Lilly, the manufacturer of Prozac, paid for a group of psychiatric "experts"—in this case psychiatrists who are strong drug proponents and often consult or do research for pharmaceutical companies—to meet in Phoenix, Arizona to discuss the growing concern about this side effect.[7] One of the main outcomes of the meeting was the decision that the term "withdrawal" should not be used for antidepressants. Instead the group proposed the euphemism "antidepressant discontinuation syndrome" to replace the term "withdrawal" in order to avoid its association with addiction.[8] After the meeting, Lilly provided financial assistance for the group of experts, many of them prominent academic psychiatrists, to publish eight papers on the antidepressant discontinuation syndrome.[9] In fact, the eight papers were bound and mailed, free of charge, to doctors across the country to help establish the term. For years the pharmaceutical industry has hidden behind the term to claim that antidepressants do not even cause symptoms of withdrawal, let alone addiction. This kind of industry spin control is part of why patients and doctors have had so much difficulty getting honest, reliable information about antidepressant withdrawal, dependence, and addiction.

Many have criticized the FDA for its alignment with the pharmaceutical industry instead of protecting the best interests of patients. When GlaxoSmithKline, in 2001, finally added a warning about Paxil withdrawal reactions to its official information on the drug, the FDA allowed the company to use the term "discontinuation" rather than "withdrawal."[10] Similarly, the FDA allows Wyeth's warning on Effexor withdrawal to use the term "discontinuation effects" rather than "withdrawal reactions."[11]

The BBC Exposé

This controversy over antidepressants being "addicting" was resolved dramatically in a British Broadcasting Corporation (BBC) two-part exposé on Paxil.[12] The first program, entitled "The Secrets of Seroxat," aired in October 2002. In May 2003, the BBC ran a follow-up program entitled "Seroxat: Emails from the Edge." Seroxat is the British name for Paxil. Hereafter, I translate the British names into their American equivalents: "The Secrets of Paxil" and "Paxil: Emails from the Edge." The response was unprecedented: The program's help line received more than 65,000 calls from viewers clamoring for more information.[13] Over 1,300 people sent emails and the BBC website received more than 120,000 hits. The overwhelming response illustrates just how big a health care crisis antidepressant withdrawal and dependence are.

The pair of programs and the flood of responses featured numerous patients who described their Paxil withdrawal in riveting detail: disabling dizziness, headaches, nausea, sweating, trembling, electric shock–like "zaps" in the brain, anxiety, crying spells, insomnia, irritability, and agitation. Many patients said antidepressant withdrawal was worse than their original psychiatric conditions. Over and over, patients said their doctors had not warned them of withdrawal side effects.

One patient featured in "The Secrets of Paxil" was Helen, a twenty-two-year-old graduate student in London. Originally prescribed Paxil for panic attacks, Helen had repeatedly tried to go off the drug without success: "I've wanted to come off it for quite a few years now but when I stopped it, I was so ill that I had to start taking it again and doctors kept telling me that it was impossible to be addicted." By the time "Paxil: Emails from the Edge" aired seven months later, Helen had finally managed to stop the drug by tapering off it painstakingly slowly. To achieve smaller and smaller doses, in the early months of the taper Helen cut Paxil pills into fragments. Eventually, the fragments became too small to be workable so she had to resort to using a dropper to administer tiny doses of Paxil in liquid form. Other patients interviewed by the BBC also referred to themselves as being "addicted" to the drug, just like my patient, Steven. Recalled one woman: "I was driving around to pharmacies begging them to give me a packet of Paxil."

In the BBC exposé, Dr. David Healy—one of Europe's leading psychiatrists—explained that patients can unwittingly become "hooked" on antidepressants.[14] David Taylor, chief pharmacist at the Maudsley Hospital in London, acknowledged that Paxil withdrawal reactions are the number one complaint of patients calling the hospital's national drug information hotline. Charles Medawar—one of the world's foremost consumer advocates on addiction to prescription drugs—said of Paxil's side effects: "I defy any scientist, any good scientist to look at the data . . . and not conclude there is a problem."[15] Richard Brook, chief executive of the mental health charity MIND, insisted: "How can we in all conscience just sit here and say it's not a problem?" And Dr. James Kennedy of the Royal College of General Practitioners advised: "It is very important to tell patients up front on Paxil and other drugs like it that there may be difficulties in coming off the drug, and that there may be at the very least a habit-forming potential with that drug in some patients."

But GlaxoSmithKline, Paxil's manufacturer, was incensed by the suggestion that antidepressants are addicting. In the first BBC show, "The Secrets of Paxil," GlaxoSmithKline's spokesman, Dr. Alastair Benbow, adamantly defended the industry's stance, insisting: "There is no reliable evidence that Paxil can cause addiction." Dr. Benbow went on to defend GlaxoSmithKline's official information for patients, which states explicitly: "Remember that you cannot become addicted to Paxil." [16] The BBC interviewer, Shelley Jofre, pressed the issue: "You're misleading them [patients]." When patients hear "remember, you cannot become addicted to Paxil," not unreasonably "many think that means they can stop taking Paxil whenever they want." One patient reacted to Dr. Benbow's denials: He's "playing on words. We shouldn't need to get dictionaries out when there are so many of us out here who are actually suffering."

In a startling turnaround, seven months later in the second BBC program, "Paxil: Emails from the Edge," GlaxoSmithKline reversed itself on the explosive issue. In response to the flood of testimonials from patients having difficulty getting off Paxil, Dr. Benbow apologetically admitted that "it's quite clear" that patients are confused by the phrase "Paxil is not addictive." Said Dr. Benbow: "That language was clearly misunderstood and therefore we have proposed that we will take out that specific wording" in the company's official information on Paxil. Indeed, shortly thereafter, GlaxoSmithKline issued a statement confirming: "We have removed all references . . . including the statement 'Paxil is not addictive.' " [17] Describing Paxil as "not addictive . . . causes confusion and may suggest to patients that Paxil treatment can be stopped abruptly," said the company.[18]

Why did GlaxoSmithKline reverse itself? The British equivalent of the FDA—the Medicines and Healthcare products Regulatory Agency—ruled that GlaxoSmithKline's spokespeople had "breached the code" that regulates company promotions when they "told journalists there was no reliable evidence that SSRIs [including Paxil] caused withdrawal symptoms or dependency." [19] Moreover, the BBC shared the unprecedented response to "The Secrets of Paxil" with GlaxoSmithKline and with the Medicines and Healthcare products Regulatory Agency, providing them with data from the 65,000 phone calls and the more than 1,300 emails. The evidence for what is commonly understood by the term "addiction" was overwhelming.

GlaxoSmithKline's May 2003 reversal is momentous and marks the turning point in the controversy over antidepressant withdrawal, dependence, and addiction. But as the BBC exposés made so clear, the controversy was more a matter of semantics than substance.[20] No one, including pharmaceutical companies, denies that antidepressants cause withdrawal reactions, although the companies quibble over what to call it and insist on the term antidepressant discontinuation syndrome. No one denies that a significant number of patients have to go back on the drugs, put the dose back up, or taper off them more slowly to obtain relief from debilitating withdrawal. The debate has centered on how to name that phenomenon. Patients stuck on an antidepressant do not say: "I'm dependent on Paxil." The technical, medical term is too awkward. Instead, patients say in plain English: "I'm addicted." As GlaxoSmithKline was forced to concede on the BBC, "addiction" is the word that patients understand when talking about the phenomenon.

In the title of the book and the title of this chapter, I use the word "addiction" in quotes because of the controversy over this term. But, having recounted how Paxil's manufacturer, GlaxoSmithKline, has reversed itself on the issue, going forward I use the term addiction the way patients use it, in plain English without quotes. I use the technical, medical term—dependence—and the laymen's term—addiction—interchangeably.

To summarize the relationship between withdrawal, dependence, and addiction, since it is central to understanding these phenomena: Withdrawal is the process of stopping or tapering off antidepressants and the characteristic symptoms that can occur as a result. Not all patients who develop withdrawal symptoms become addicted, or dependent. Addiction occurs when patients suffer such intolerable or incapacitating withdrawal symptoms that they are forced to restart the drugs, put the dose back up, or taper off them more slowly. Patients are then dependent on the antidepressants for as long as it takes to wean off the drugs. Dependence and addiction are the same things: dependence being the technical, medical term used by doctors and addiction the plain English term used by patients or found in dictionaries like the *Oxford English Dictionary*.[21] Because clarifying the terms "withdrawal," "dependence," and "addiction" is so important, Table 2.1 summarizes the terminology.

Table 2.1 TERMINOLOGY OF ANTIDEPRESSANT
WITHDRAWAL, DEPENDENCE, AND ADDICTION

TERM	DEFINITION
Withdrawal	The process of stopping or tapering off antidepressants and the characteristic symptoms that can develop as a result.
Addiction and Dependence *(These are interchangeable terms: Addiction is the plain English term while dependence is the technical, medical term.)*	Patients suffering such uncomfortable or incapacitating withdrawal symptoms that they are forced to restart antidepressants, put the dose back up, or taper off them more slowly. Patients are dependent, or addicted, to antidepressants for as long as it takes to wean off them.

3

The Withdrawal Spectrum
Mild, Moderate, and Severe Withdrawal Reactions

John: A Case of Paxil Withdrawal with Severe Consequences

"Cambridge Police. Open up. You're under arrest," shouted the uniformed officers as they banged on the door to John's room in the Sheraton Commander Hotel in Harvard Square.

"The police?" John, startled, lunged out of bed and nearly crashed to the floor in the darkened room because of severe dizziness caused by Paxil withdrawal. "How could they have found me here?" Switching on the lights, John steadied himself against the wall. His head felt swollen and achy, like he had water sloshing around in his brain. Flu-like aches and pains wracked his body. Tingling sensations raced down both arms into his hands. John felt faint, like throwing up, he was so nauseous.

"Open up. Cambridge police." The officers continued to pound heavily. A Harvard College student, John was suffering from severe Paxil withdrawal, whose symptoms included impulsivity and poor judgment. Just hours before the police arrived, John had impulsively stolen the backpack of a fellow student. After the theft, dazed and confused, he took refuge in the hotel room, paying with a charge card he found in the stolen backpack. My life is ruined, thought John, his head spinning as he pulled on his clothes.

"You're under arrest." The police kept banging on the door. Although a hotel security guard had unlocked the door, John had fastened the chain lock on the inside before going to sleep. As a result, the door opened only a few inches. As the police shouted and banged the door against the chain, John dressed as quickly as he could to meet the policemen's demands.

"I'm coming," shouted John as he moved toward the door. The police backed off briefly to allow him to release the chain lock. The police had no way of knowing John was a student in the throes of antidepressant withdrawal whose behavior was completely out of character. At six foot four inches and 225 pounds, John cut a formidable figure. Taking him for a potential criminal, the police rushed John. John's bewildered protests were lost in the melee. "I was overtaken by four police officers," says John reflecting on his ordeal. "It was the most terrifying experience of my life."

I first met John a month after he was arrested and criminal charges were brought against him. He was referred to me because of my interest in antidepressant withdrawal. At the time, John was in his junior year at Harvard. For more than a year and a half after his arrest, the resulting legal proceedings and disciplinary hearings threatened his degree and future career. He could have been expelled from college. He nearly lost a coveted job. And he spent months weaning off Paxil. John gave me permission to tell his story because he wants doctors and patients to be aware that antidepressant withdrawal can have severe, lasting repercussions in people's lives.

After his sophomore year in college, John had taken a year off to work in Washington, D.C. John was first prescribed Paxil by a family doctor in Washington in the spring before he returned to Harvard. He went to see the doctor not because he was depressed or anxious but because he was planning a trip to Jamaica with friends before returning to school and needed travel immunizations. During the course of the fifteen-minute travel clinic appointment, John mentioned being "apprehensive" about returning to the role of a student after working full-time for a year. The doctor, who had never met John before, immediately offered him Paxil, at a dose of 20 milligrams a day, saying it would calm any anxieties he had about returning to school. Says John in retrospect: "What could he have been thinking? I wasn't depressed. I wasn't panicking. I was mildly anxious about returning to the role of a student. What I was feeling was perfectly normal."

John was reluctant to go on medication but the doctor pressed him, advising that if he didn't, the anxiety could get worse. "I was taught to respect authority figures, so I went along with him," says John. "He gave me a hepatitis vaccine for the trip and I had to return for the second shot. If I hadn't had to go back, I might never have gone on the Paxil. But because I had to report back to the doctor, I didn't want to tell him I hadn't taken the Paxil."

Not only did the doctor start John on Paxil, he wrote prescriptions for many months worth of refills. As a result, John was on Paxil unsupervised through his trip to Jamaica, the remainder of the summer, his move from Washington to Cambridge, and the beginning of his first semester back in school.

John's transition back to school went more smoothly than he had expected. He found he was a more disciplined student, made many new friends, and began a relationship with a new girlfriend. One Saturday in late October, six months after starting Paxil, John noticed he was running low on the medication and needed to go to the pharmacy to pick up another month's supply. But because he was doing so well, he decided instead to go off the medication. He took his last dose on Saturday morning, innocently thinking nothing of it. Since he had not been warned about Paxil withdrawal, it did not occur to John that he needed medical supervision to stop the drug. The dose John had been taking, 20 milligrams a day, is a standard recommended dose of Paxil.

By Monday John thought he had a severe case of the flu. His muscles and joints were aching and painful. He felt nauseous and dizzy. Overcome with malaise, he had difficulty concentrating in class and keeping up with his homework. John thought he had the chills because of the strange tingling sensations shooting down both his arms. He talked by phone with his mother, who agreed he must have the flu. In fact, John was in Paxil withdrawal.

John pushed himself to keep going to his classes, but as the week went on he felt worse and worse. By Wednesday he could hardly get out of bed. Finally, on Thursday he felt so ill and dizzy at the end of his math class that he could not get out of the chair to leave the room. "I couldn't stand up. I felt like I was going to pass out," says John. As the classroom emptied, John's professor noticed him slumped in the chair. Discovering that John felt too ill to get up from his seat, the professor called the medical clinic. The clinic dispatched a nurse who, along with the professor, assisted John to the clinic for treatment.

One of the family doctors at the clinic evaluated John. Although John appeared to have a severe case of the flu, as part of a thorough evaluation, she asked if John was on any medication. Fortunately, John mentioned that he had recently stopped Paxil. Equally fortunately, the doctor knew something about antidepressant withdrawal.

The doctor told John he was suffering from Paxil withdrawal. John was dumbfounded. The doctor instructed him to go back on the medication to treat the withdrawal. At a later date he could consult with a psychiatrist about tapering more slowly off the drug. John left the clinic stunned and still reeling from his severe Paxil withdrawal reaction.

Shortly after leaving the clinic, still in acute withdrawal and feeling highly agitated and irritable, John impulsively stole the backpack of a fellow student. "I don't know what came over me." John shakes his head in retrospect. "I felt like a zombie. I grabbed the backpack and ran off with it in full view of other people. I understand now that my impulsivity was caused by Paxil withdrawal. But at the time, my own behavior was baffling to me." As surprising as John's behavior may seem, antidepressant withdrawal reactions published in medical journals include reports of impulsive, aggressive behavior, like shoplifting and physical assaults.[1]

Inside the backpack, John found the other student's wallet, ID, charge cards, and money. Posing as the student, he checked into a hotel because he felt so ill, frightened, and in need of somewhere to take refuge. The police tracked John through his use of the charge cards and arrested him. He was taken to the police station, where he was booked with "larceny" for stealing the credit card and with using a "false document" for pretending to be the student whose credit card he stole. Because the theft occurred on Harvard property, the university police and administration also became involved. John was in trouble not only with the law, he was in trouble with the disciplinary board of Harvard College.

The day after John's arrest, all of the withdrawal symptoms vanished because he resumed the Paxil: "I felt clear as a bell. The dizziness, nausea, aches and pains . . . everything was gone. I could think clearly. My energy was back. It was amazing." Unfortunately for John his problems had only just begun: "I woke up bright and alert to the nightmare of what I had done." John's behavior while in the throes of Paxil withdrawal was completely out of character. He had no prior police record. Nor had he ever had any disciplinary problems. He had always been a thoughtful, considerate, law-abiding citizen.

John immediately apologized and made restitution to the student whose backpack he stole. A month after his arrest, he had his first hearing before a judge who set a date for John's case to go to trial in the spring. At around this time, John was referred to me. He was on Paxil an additional four months until a gradual taper allowed him to wean off it. Despite the pain and suffering he endured with the legal proceedings and threats to his career, John managed well without the drug once he weaned himself off it. John went through the entire ordeal without ever telling his family. His parents were not well off and he felt they had neither the personal nor financial resources to help him. He feared that if he told his parents they would be devastated. His younger brothers and sisters looked up to him as a role model, which, for the family's sake, he did not want to jeopardize.

In January, John took his semester exams with the added stress of the legal proceedings and of not knowing whether he would ultimately be allowed to finish his degree at Harvard. Fortunately, because of the medical records documenting his Paxil withdrawal, the judge eventually dismissed the criminal charges against him. Following the judge's example, Harvard eventually took no disciplinary action.

But John's troubles were still not over. At the end of the academic year, a sought-after summer job he had been offered at a consulting firm was rescinded when the firm found out about his difficulties with the law, even though they had already been resolved in his favor. Together, one of the school's career counselors and I lobbied the firm intensively to reinstate John's summer position. Initially, our efforts seemed to be in vain: the hiring partner denied our request. Finally, the career counselor threatened to reevaluate the firm's recruiting at Harvard if this was the way they would treat someone in John's circumstances. At this point, the firm backed down. I remember the career counselor reporting the good news but noting: "We were probably only able to save John's hide because we're Harvard and because of the clout that allowed us to bring to bear."

John did extremely well at the summer job. The following year, as a senior, he landed an excellent job in another consulting firm that was to begin after he graduated. He thought his problems were behind him. But, as graduation approached, he had to fill out routine employment forms for the new firm. One question asked if John had ever been arrested. He answered honestly and innocently explained the circumstances. A week later, the nightmare had returned: the firm announced they had to do a thorough evaluation of whether they could honor their offer of employment. Once again, he spent weeks getting documentation from everyone involved in the incident, including a letter from the math professor who found him ill in the classroom, the medical records of the doctor who diagnosed the Paxil withdrawal, and a letter from me. Almost up until the time he graduated, John was unsure whether he had a job. Fortunately, the firm made the right decision in the end, honoring their employment offer after reviewing his case.

John's pain and suffering—the severe withdrawal symptoms, being arrested, having to go back on Paxil to slowly wean off, and enduring the legal proceedings, disciplinary hearings, and threats to his career—lasted more than a year and a half. In retrospect, it is doubtful he even needed Paxil in the first place. His "worries" about going back to school never warranted prescribing Paxil.

Notice a common theme in Diana's, Steven's, and John's cases: antidepressant withdrawal reactions cause considerable pain and suffering for many patients. Diana was dependent on Zoloft, took the antidepressant for four more years than she needed it, and endured significant weight gain and severe sexual side effects that negatively affected her marriage. Steven felt like a "Paxil junkie" and was forced to wean off Paxil over the course of months because he was unable to stop it cold turkey the way he had stopped smoking cigarettes. John's being arrested while in Paxil withdrawal will probably haunt him for the rest of his life, as he will continue to have to report it on his job applications and in other circumstances. Still, the consequences of John's Paxil withdrawal could have been even worse. What if his math professor had not lingered after class, noticed how sick John was, and brought him to the medical clinic? When the doctor in the clinic asked John if he was on any medication, what if he had simply answered "No"? John mentioned that he had recently stopped Paxil by chance, not because he thought there was any connection to how sick he was feeling. And what if the doctor, like many, had not known much about antidepressant withdrawal? If no one had figured out that John was in Paxil withdrawal, then the consequences of his behavior would have been far worse. He would have been blamed for the theft, probably been expelled from college, lost his job, and truly had his life ruined. How many people have had these kinds of serious consequences of antidepressant withdrawal? Like most patients, Diana, Steven, and John were not warned about antidepressant withdrawal reactions let alone told how severe the reactions and their consequences can be.

Symptoms of Antidepressant Withdrawal

To prevent the kind of reactions Diana, Steven, and John suffered, patients and doctors need to be well informed about the symptoms of antidepressant withdrawal. Impulsivity and poor judgment are just two of more than fifty symptoms that have been identified in published case reports and large-scale, systematic studies of the phenomenon.[2] The complete list of symptoms can be found in Table 3.1. Notice in the table that withdrawal symptoms are divided into two major categories: *psychiatric symptoms* and *medical symptoms*. Distinguishing between these two categories is critical to recognizing antidepressant withdrawal reactions and to differentiating them from other medical and psychiatric conditions. Patients can have any mix of psychiatric and medical withdrawal symptoms. In John's case, his psychiatric withdrawal symptoms were poor judgment and impulsivity, whereas his medical withdrawal symptoms were dizziness, the sensation of water sloshing around in his head, flu-like aches and pains, tingling sensations in his arms, and nausea.

The discussion of psychiatric and medical antidepressant withdrawal symptoms that follows applies in particular to two classes of today's popular antidepressants: the selective serotonin reuptake inhibitors (SSRIs)—Paxil, Zoloft, Celexa, Lexapro, Prozac, and Luvox—and the closely related serotonin and noradrenalin reuptake inhibitors (SNRIs)—Effexor, Cymbalta, and Serzone. The two remaining antidepressants, Remeron and Wellbutrin, are discussed later in the chapter.

Psychiatric Symptoms of Antidepressant Withdrawal

The psychiatric symptoms of antidepressant withdrawal are not a return of the patient's underlying psychiatric condition. Rather, they are drug-induced withdrawal phenomena. Later in the chapter I describe how to distinguish psychiatric withdrawal symptoms from the patient's original psychiatric condition. But first, one needs to be familiar with the full range of withdrawal symptoms.

Notice in Table 3.1 that the psychiatric symptoms of antidepressant withdrawal can mimic depression and anxiety, the two most common conditions for which the drugs are prescribed. Virtually all the common

Table 3.1 SYMPTOMS OF ANTIDEPRESSANT WITHDRAWAL

PSYCHIATRIC SYMPTOMS	MEDICAL SYMPTOMS
That Mimic Depression	*That Mimic the Flu*
1. Crying spells	29. Flu-like aches and pains
2. Worsened mood	30. Fever
3. Low energy (fatigue, lethargy, malaise)	31. Sweats
4. Trouble concentrating	32. Chills
5. Insomnia or trouble sleeping	33. Runny nose
6. Change in appetite	34. Sore eyes
7. Suicidal thoughts	
8. Suicide attempts	*That Mimic Gastroenteritis*
	35. Nausea
That Mimic Anxiety Disorders	36. Vomiting
9. Anxious, nervous, tense	37. Diarrhea
10. Panic attacks (racing heart, breathless)	38. Abdominal pain or cramps
11. Chest pain	39. Stomach bloating
12. Trembling, jittery, or shaking	
	Dizziness
Irritability and Aggression	40. Disequilibrium
13. Irritability	41. Spinning, swaying, lightheaded
14. Agitation (restlessness, hyperactivity)	42. Hung over or waterlogged feeling
15. Impulsivity	43. Unsteady gait, poor coordination
16. Aggressiveness	44. Motion sickness
17. Self-harm	
18. Homicidal thoughts or urges	*Headache*
	45. Headache
Confusion and Memory Problems	
19. Confusion or cognitive difficulties	*Tremor*
20. Memory problems or forgetfulness	46. Tremor
Mood Swings	*Sensory Abnormalities*
21. Elevated mood (feeling high)	47. Numbness, burning, or tingling
22. Mood swings	48. Electric zap–like sensations in the brain
23. Manic-like reactions	49. Electric shock–like sensations in the body
	50. Abnormal visual sensations
Hallucinations	51. Ringing or other noises in the ears
24. Auditory hallucinations	52. Abnormal smells or tastes
25. Visual hallucinations	
	Other
Dissociation	53. Drooling or excessive saliva
26. Feeling detached or unreal	54. Slurred speech
	55. Blurred vision
Other	56. Muscle cramps, stiffness, twitches
27. Excessive or intense dreaming	57. Feeling of restless legs
28. Nightmares	58. Uncontrollable twitching of mouth

symptoms of depression are also symptoms of antidepressant withdrawal: crying, sadness, worsened mood, low energy, inability to concentrate, disturbed sleep, change in appetite, suicidal thoughts, and suicide attempts. Experts note that the crying spells are "dramatic and disappear quickly" when the antidepressant is reintroduced.[3] The worsened mood can result in severe, paralyzing sadness. The low energy is described as "lethargy," "malaise," "apathy," and "asthenia," a psychiatric term for feeling weak.[4] Patients may have difficulty concentrating.[5] Both increased and decreased appetite have been reported.[6] Insomnia is the most common sleep disturbance.[7] Some patients fall asleep without difficulty but sleep fitfully, waking up repeatedly during the night. Excessive dreaming, vivid dreams, and nightmares can also occur.[8] The dreams are often frightening ones involving harm to oneself or harm to others.[9]

In severe antidepressant withdrawal reactions, patients can become suicidal and homicidal.[10] Researchers at the National Institute of Mental Health reported in the British medical journal *The Lancet* on a patient in severe Paxil withdrawal who "became preoccupied with homicidal thoughts and plans, initially directed towards acquaintances and later towards his own children. These became so intense and ego-dystonic [alien and distressing to the patient] that he contemplated suicide."[11] In another case reported in the journal *Human Psychopharmacology*, a thirty-six-year-old woman had a "severe [Zoloft] withdrawal reaction of vertigo [the sensation of rooms spinning], dizziness, ataxia [lack of coordinated movement], nausea, diplopia [double vision], heaviness in her head and a feeling of dissociation [an out-of-body experience in which one feels outside oneself, observing oneself]. Her only relief was lying flat on her back in bed."[12] After nine days of such severe symptoms, the patient took an overdose of sleeping pills in a suicide attempt. She was hospitalized and not released from the hospital until "the withdrawal reactions had subsided." Patients who have such severe withdrawal reactions can become psychologically stuck on their antidepressant because they are too frightened to go down on the dose again after experiencing traumatizing withdrawal side effects. In a June 10, 2003, "Dear Doctor" letter, GlaxoSmithKline reported that children and adolescents under the age of eighteen may be particularly vulnerable to becoming suicidal during withdrawal.[13] GlaxoSmithKline reported that in the company's studies, children and adolescents tapering off Paxil frequently developed withdrawal symptoms of "crying, mood fluctuations, self-harm, suicidal thoughts, and attempted suicide." In March 2004, the FDA issued its warning that adult and pediatric patients may become suicidal when they decrease the dose of their antidepressants while tapering off the drugs.[14] Because patients' becoming suicidal when they change the dose of anti-depressants is such a serious side effect, the next chapter discusses this phenomenon in greater detail.

Withdrawal-induced anxiety is described in reports published in medical journals as "nervousness," "jitteriness," "panic attacks," "palpitations [racing heartbeats]," "shaking," and "feeling tense."[15] Patients in antidepressant withdrawal feel "fragile," like they have little reserve to cope with life's demands.

The irritability of antidepressant withdrawal can be strikingly like the irritability people experience when they stop smoking cigarettes.[16] Some patients stopping antidepressants describe wanting to punch walls. Irritability can lead to agitation, restlessness, hyperactivity, impulsivity, and aggression. Completely out of character, impulsive behavior can include destroying objects, "explosive vocal outbursts," "tantrums," "physical fights," and "shoplifting."[17] Some patients engage in self-injurious behavior, like punching walls or cutting themselves.[18]

Patients in antidepressant withdrawal can find such out-of-character feelings and behavior "unbearably distressing."[19] So, too can family members trying to cope with the sudden changes in behavior. "I tried not to take his short temper and rudeness personally," said the wife of one patient of mine, "because I knew he was in withdrawal. But it was hard. He's not normally like that and I wouldn't normally put up with being treated that way." The behavioral changes are even more upsetting to families when they do not know the cause is antidepressant withdrawal.

Patients who have cognitive difficulties as a result of antidepressant withdrawal can become confused or have memory problems.[20] Less common but at times quite serious psychiatric symptoms of withdrawal include auditory and visual hallucinations;[21] manic-like or unstable, rapidly changing moods;[22] and feeling detached or unreal.[23] These severe psychiatric withdrawal symptoms are discussed in greater detail in the next chapter.

Medical Symptoms of Antidepressant Withdrawal

The medical symptoms of antidepressant withdrawal can mimic a variety of medical conditions. Dizziness, poor coordination, and unsteady gait can be mistaken for a stroke, cardiac event, or inner ear problem.[24] Flu-like aches and pains, fever, sweats, and chills can be mistaken for the flu.[25] And nausea, vomiting, diarrhea, bloating, and stomach cramps can be mistaken for a "stomach bug."

Repeated studies have found dizziness the most common medical symptom of antidepressant withdrawal.[26] In reports published in medical journals, patients describe the dizziness in a variety of ways: "disequilibrium," "unsteadiness," "swaying," "spinning," "lightheadedness," "spaced out," "swimming," "water logged," "water sloshing around in my head," "drunken," or "buzzing."[27]

Movement—such as walking, climbing stairs, turning one's head, or just moving one's eyes—often exacerbates the dizziness.[28] A patient may say she has been dizzy but feels fine sitting in the doctor's office. Simply asking the patient to turn her head while remaining seated often brings the dizziness on again. The dizziness of antidepressant withdrawal has been compared to motion, or car, sickness.[29] Because of unsteady gait, patients may have difficulty walking up stairs or they may bump into furniture.[30]

Withdrawal-induced dizziness can have a profound effect on patients' day-to-day lives, making it difficult to do everything from driving a car to walking around. If the dizziness is severe, the only way to relieve it may be sitting or lying still.[31] When this occurs, patients can be incapacitated and miss days of work or school.[32]

The headaches of antidepressant withdrawal can be debilitating.[33] The headaches may be throbbing or dull, diffuse or localized. Patients often use over-the-counter medications like Tylenol to blunt antidepressant headaches.

Withdrawal-induced tremors are distressing to many patients because they associate tremors with serious drug addiction. The best way for a doctor to observe the severity of tremors is to have patients hold both their arms and hands outstretched in front of them.

Sensory abnormalities are among the more bizarre medical symptoms of antidepressant withdrawal.[34] These include tingling, burning, and electric shock–like sensations. In one of the most frightening sensory disturbances, patients describe electric zap–like sensations in their brains. These are lightning-like jolts inside the head that make patients feel as if they are having a dangerous neurological event such as a stroke.[35] Alternatively, electric shock–like sensations can occur in the body, especially the legs and the area around the mouth.[36] In some patients withdrawing from antidepressants, bending the neck brings on waves of electric shock–like sensations down the spine, arms, and legs.[37] Any of these sensations can be quite frightening to patients, who worry that antidepressant withdrawal may be injuring their nervous system. Unfortunately, we do not have a good explanation for why antidepressant withdrawal can cause these often startling symptoms.

In other patients, burning or tingling sensations radiate, or "shoot," down the arms or through the body. Abnormal visual phenomena include flashing lights, "jerking" or "jumping" vision, and geometric shapes.[38] Ringing in the ears or other noises, like swishing sounds, may also occur.[39]

Less common, but at times quite distressing, medical symptoms of antidepressant withdrawal include drooling because of excessive saliva, difficulty speaking clearly because of slurred speech, chest pain, muscle twitching or spasms, muscle cramps or stiffness, restless legs, and uncontrollable twitching of the mouth.[40]

Other Antidepressants

The above discussion is based on published reports of antidepressant withdrawal reactions with two closely related classes of today's popular antidepressants: selective serotonin reuptake inhibitors (SSRIs) and serotonin and noradrenalin reuptake inhibitors (SNRIs). Two of today's popular antidepressants do not fall into either of these classes: Remeron and Wellbutrin.

Remeron boosts serotonin and noradrenalin by a different mechanism from the SSRIs and SNRIs.[41] The details of Remeron's mechanism of action are unimportant for our purposes. Because Remeron boosts serotonin and noradrenalin, the withdrawal symptoms seen with Remeron resemble those seen with SSRIs and SNRIs.[42]

Wellbutrin boosts a different brain chemical, called dopamine.[43] Wellbutrin is also marketed under a different name, Zyban, for smoking cessation.[44] Because Wellbutrin/Zyban boosts dopamine, withdrawal reactions look somewhat different from withdrawal reactions with drugs that boost serotonin. There are few published cases of Wellbutrin/Zyban withdrawal reactions.[45] But in my experience, irritability is a more prominent feature of withdrawal reactions in patients stopping Wellbutrin/Zyban than in patients stopping other antidepressants. Indeed, patients withdrawing from Wellbutrin/Zyban look remarkably like people withdrawing from cigarettes, which may not be so surprising since

Wellbutrin/Zyban is used to treat nicotine withdrawal. Patients withdrawing from Wellbutrin/Zyban can become so irritable that they feel like punching walls. They can be quite abrupt, rude, hostile, and aggressive with spouses and friends, as well as with strangers. Of course, irritability, hostility, and aggression are also withdrawal side effects of antidepressants that boost serotonin. But they are more commonly the most prominent withdrawal symptoms with Wellbutrin/Zyban.

Distinguishing Psychiatric Symptoms of Withdrawal from Depressive Relapse

The fact that the psychiatric symptoms of withdrawal can mimic depressive relapse requires doctors to distinguish between the two. In most instances, the psychiatric symptoms of withdrawal can be distinguished from relapse relatively easily *so long as doctors and patients know what to look for* to make the distinction. The features setting psychiatric symptoms of withdrawal apart from depressive relapse are:

- Timing of the onset of symptoms
- Presence of medical symptoms of withdrawal
- Characteristic time course for the symptoms to peak and fade
- Dramatic disappearance of the symptoms if the drug is reinstated

The Timing of the Onset of Symptoms

Psychiatric symptoms of withdrawal appear abruptly within days to weeks of stopping an antidepressant, lowering the dose, or forgetting to take a few doses. In one study of Paxil withdrawal, symptoms appeared within four days in 86 percent of cases.[46] The close temporal relationship between stopping the drugs and developing symptoms is characteristic of withdrawal.[47] By contrast, depressive relapse occurs gradually one to two months or more after stopping an antidepressant.[48]

The Presence of Medical Symptoms of Withdrawal

Patients often panic when thrown into antidepressant withdrawal because they think their original psychiatric condition has suddenly reappeared. Distraught over the psychiatric symptoms of withdrawal, patients can easily overlook medical symptoms like dizziness, headaches, nausea, flu-like aches and pains, and sensory abnormalities like burning or tingling sensations, especially if they are not too severe.

Doctors need to specifically ask if any medical symptoms of withdrawal are present. Often dizziness—the most common medical symptom—provides an important clue that the patient is, in fact, in antidepressant withdrawal. The doctor needs to inquire systematically, reviewing all the symptoms of withdrawal to be sure none are overlooked. In contrast to withdrawal, depressive relapse does not include medical symptoms such as dizziness, nausea, headaches, flu-like aches and pains, or sensory abnormalities like burning, tingling, or electric shock–like sensations.

Patients should be reassured that the psychiatric symptoms of withdrawal are not a reappearance of their original psychiatric condition. Even GlaxoSmithKline acknowledges: "Such symptoms [i.e., withdrawal symptoms] should not be interpreted as indicating a worsening of the psychiatric illness being treated."[49] Rather, says GlaxoSmithKline, "symptoms usually start abruptly within a few days of [Paxil] discontinuation and can be distinguished from relapse symptoms, which occur later and build up gradually."[50]

Characteristic Time Course for the Symptoms to Peak and Fade

Following a small dosage reduction, if the patient is able to wait and see—to tolerate a mild to moderate antidepressant withdrawal reaction—the symptoms typically peak within seven to ten days and clear over the course of two to three weeks. By contrast, relapse does not clear in two to three weeks. Depression is typically ongoing and may get progressively worse. According to the American Psychiatric Association's *Diagnostic and Statistical Manual of Mental Disorders (DSM)*—the profession's diagnostic bible—to officially diagnose clinical depression a patient's symptoms must be present for a minimum of two weeks.[51] When patients are able to tolerate mild to moderate antidepressant withdrawal reactions, by two weeks the symptoms have often clearly improved and may have already disappeared.

Dramatic Disappearance of the Symptoms If the Drug Is Reinstated

When an antidepressant is restarted to suppress a withdrawal reaction, the symptoms begin to clear within hours and often completely disappear within twenty-four hours.[52] If ambiguity exists over whether or not the patient is in withdrawal, the patient can take a "test dose" of the antidepressant to see if the symptoms clear quickly. The test dose should be the dose the patient was previously taking. If the patient's symptoms disappear within one day, this clearly indicates the patient was in withdrawal. By contrast, when a patient relapses, an antidepressant takes two to four weeks to work, although side effects of the drug can appear sooner.[53] In many published cases, patients repeatedly go back on antidepressants to suppress intolerable withdrawal only to have the withdrawal symptoms recur like clockwork if the patient again tries to go off the drug, clearly establishing an on-again, off-again cause-and-effect relationship.[54]

Thus antidepressant withdrawal—like all drug withdrawal—is fairly stereotypical, making it relatively easy to recognize because of a characteristic pattern of symptoms, onset, peak, time course, and dramatic disappearance in response to resuming the drug. As a result, in the vast majority of cases physicians and patients can easily distinguish withdrawal reactions from relapse. Since distinguishing the psychiatric symptoms of withdrawal from depressive relapse is so important, the differences are summarized in Table 3.2 for easy reference.

Distinguishing Medical Symptoms of Withdrawal from Other Medical Conditions

Just as the psychiatric symptoms of antidepressant withdrawal can mimic a patient's original psychiatric condition, so too the medical symptoms of antidepressant withdrawal can be confused with other medical conditions. This occurs when doctors do not know about antidepressant withdrawal and therefore do not consider it as an explanation for the patient's symptoms. Patients in antidepressant withdrawal may call their doctors' offices for reassurance, visit the doctors' offices for urgent medical attention, or go to hospital emergency departments. Expensive medical tests and treatments may be ordered.[55] The patient's "illness" can remain a mystery unless a doctor is eventually consulted who knows about antidepressant withdrawal and accurately diagnoses it.

Given the wide variety of medical symptoms of antidepressant withdrawal, a patient's condition can be confused with numerous medical conditions. A few examples published in medical journals include:

• A man admitted to Massachusetts General Hospital in Boston because he was thought to be having a heart attack.[56] Describing the man's case in 1997 in the *Journal of Clinical Psychiatry*, Dr. Jerrold Rosenbaum reported that after the patient was hospitalized, "it

Table 3.2 DISTINGUISHING PSYCHIATRIC SYMPTOMS OF WITHDRAWAL FROM DEPRESSIVE RELAPSE

TEST	WITHDRAWAL	RELAPSE
Is the onset of symptoms abrupt over days to a week?	Withdrawal occurs abruptly within days to weeks of stopping an antidepressant, lowering the dose, or forgetting to take a few doses.	Relapse symptoms occur one to two months or more after stopping an antidepressant and develop gradually.
Are characteristic medical symptoms of withdrawal present?	Characteristic medical symptoms of withdrawal include dizziness, headaches, nausea, flu-like aches and pains, and sensory abnormalities, such as burning, tingling, or other abnormal sensations. (Note: The patient may have overlooked these symptoms while focusing on the psychiatric withdrawal symptoms.)	The characteristic medical symptoms of withdrawal are not present in depressive relapse.
Do the symptoms peak and clear in the time course typical of withdrawal reactions?	If the patient "toughs out" tolerable withdrawal symptoms, the symptoms usually peak within seven to ten days and clear within two to three weeks.	Depressive relapse does not spontaneously clear in two to three weeks. Relapse continues, and may get worse.
Do the symptoms disappear quickly if the patient is given a test dose of the antidepressant?	Given a test dose, a patient's withdrawal symptoms quickly disappear within 24 hours, clearly indicating that the patient was having a withdrawal reaction.	When a patient relapses, an antidepressant takes 2 to 4 weeks to work to treat depression. (Side effects of the drug can, however, appear sooner.)

turned out that the symptoms occurred in the context of Effexor" withdrawal. When the Effexor was restarted, his symptoms cleared.

- A young New York woman who stopped 40 milligrams a day of Prozac developed eye twitching and "extreme" dizziness that caused her to fall into furniture.[57] Her case was reported in the *American Journal of Psychiatry* in August 1995. The report stated: "Examination by a neurologist and an otorhinolaryngologist [ear, nose, and throat specialist], a magnetic resonance imaging of the head [an MRI brain scan], and tests for Lyme [tick] disease" were conducted before the symptoms were recognized as Prozac withdrawal and suppressed by restarting the drug.

- A forty-five-year-old man in Fort Sill, Oklahoma developed left-sided facial numbness and blurred vision several days after stopping 20 milligrams a day of Paxil.[58] His case was reported in the April 2000 issue of the *Journal of Clinical Psychopharmacology*. According to the report, the patient was referred by his family doctor to the vascular surgery department, where he had an ultrasound of the arteries in his neck and X-rays of his spine. When his symptoms remained a mystery, he was sent to a neurosurgeon and had brain and spinal MRI scans. He was then sent to a cardiologist for a Holter monitor, a twenty-four-hour EKG looking for irregular heartbeats. He was referred to a neurologist who was once again unable to diagnose his symptoms. All of the tests came back normal and the patient's symptoms peaked and cleared before any of the doctors made the connection to stopping Paxil. The connection was only made two years later when he went back on Paxil and then developed the same withdrawal symptoms when he stopped it again.

- A thirty-nine-year-old woman in treatment at the Louisiana State University School of Medicine in Shreveport stopped 20 milligrams a day of Paxil when she "ran out of medication" while on vacation.[59] Her case was reported in the *Journal of Clinical Psychopharmacology* in October 1996. The patient "decided not to continue it because she felt that she was doing well" after a year on the drug. A day after stopping Paxil, she developed nausea, hot and cold flashes, headaches, lightheadedness, and waves of "electrical shocks going through her back and limbs. . . . Over the next 2 days, her symptoms increased markedly. The sensations of electrical shock became so severe with movement that she began sitting as still as possible." Eventually, she interrupted her vacation to go to the nearest hospital emergency department. The doctor who examined her there found that bending her "neck produced sensations of electrical shock down the spine and along the limbs." The symptoms were "almost disabling" because the patient felt so uncomfortable that she could not walk or move. The waves of electric shock sensations triggered by the patient's bending her neck were diagnosed as "identical to Lhermitte's sign [which is characteristically] seen with dysfunction of the posterior spinal cord" in neurological diseases. Fortunately, the connection was made between the symptoms and the patient stopping Paxil three days earlier. When the patient was restarted on Paxil, her symptoms improved within four hours and she was subsequently able to taper off the drug "with only minor symptomatology."

- A thirty-nine-year-old woman from Halifax, Canada stopped 40 milligrams a day of Paxil after taking the drug for a year.[60] Her case was reported in the *Journal of Psychopharmacology* in 2001. Two weeks after stopping Paxil, she developed a prominent "tremor of her hands, shock-like sensations and weakness and numbness in her hands and legs" which felt worse on her left side. When the patient's psychiatrist failed to diagnose her symptoms as Paxil withdrawal, she went to a hospital emergency department where a neurologist hospitalized her fearing that she had had a stroke. The patient had a CAT scan of her brain and an EEG. When the tests came back normal, she eventually consulted a new psychiatrist who accurately diagnosed the Paxil withdrawal reaction. The patient's symptoms persisted for eight weeks after she stopped the drug.

To prevent these unnecessary, wasteful scenarios that take a heavy toll on patients and the health care system, doctors need to be well informed about how to diagnose and manage antidepressant withdrawal reactions. Patients seeking urgent or emergency medical care are routinely asked what medications they are on. But, in addition, they need to be asked if they have recently stopped an antidepressant, lowered the dose, or accidentally missed a few doses, all of which can produce withdrawal reactions.

Common Symptoms of Antidepressant Withdrawal

In order to accurately recognize, or diagnose, antidepressant withdrawal, one needs to be well informed about the full range of withdrawal symptoms. At the same time, it is helpful to know the most common scenarios, or clusters of symptoms, of antidepressant withdrawal.[61] Common scenarios are:

- *Patients with predominantly psychiatric symptoms.* These patients typically have some combination of anxiety, crying spells, fatigue, irritability, and agitation, the most common psychiatric symptoms of antidepressant withdrawal. The panic patients experience if they mistake withdrawal symptoms for a return of their original psychiatric condition is greatly compounded if their doctors are not informed or are ill-informed about antidepressant withdrawal and make the same mistake, "confirming" the patient's worst fear. Typically these patients are also dizzy or have other medical symptoms of withdrawal but they have not paid attention to the medical symptoms because they are so preoccupied with the psychiatric symptoms.

- *Patients with predominantly medical symptoms.* The most common medical symptom is dizziness. Other common scenarios are flu-like syndromes, gastrointestinal symptoms, or headaches. Patients who appear to have severe cases of the flu will have generalized aches and pains, sometimes accompanied by fever, sweats, and chills. Patients who look like they have a severe stomach "bug" will have nausea, vomiting, and diarrhea. These patients often feel dizzy, fatigued, and quite ill. They may go to their doctors' offices for urgent care appointments or to hospital emergency rooms. Sometimes they are dehydrated and require intravenous fluids because they have not been taking in enough liquids. Typically, these patients also feel anxious, tired, and fragile but their focus is the medical symptoms, because they feel so physically ill. Some patients are driven to urgent care appointments or emergency rooms by withdrawal headaches. Often they have tried over-the-counter remedies that did not work to alleviate the headaches. When questioned in detail, these patients, too, often have other symptoms like dizziness, anxiety, irritability, or insomnia, but their focus is the splitting headaches.

Table 3.3 GLOBAL ASSESSMENT OF THE SEVERITY
OF ANTIDEPRESSANT WITHDRAWAL REACTIONS

SEVERITY	CRITERIA
Mild withdrawal	Presence of: • Withdrawal symptoms (from Table 3.1) that are tolerated relatively comfortably and do not affect one's ability to function normally
Moderate withdrawal	Presence of: • Withdrawal symptoms (from Table 3.1) that are uncomfortable and negatively affect, even to a minimal degree, one's ability to think clearly and/or function normally
Severe withdrawal	Presence of one or more debilitating or alarming withdrawal symptoms (from Table 3.1) that: • include suicidal thoughts, suicidal behavior, harm to oneself or others, hallucinations, or manic-like symptoms • make it impossible to function normally for all or part of the day • require putting the dose of the antidepressant back up after a dosage reduction • require restarting the antidepressant if it had been stopped altogether • require tapering the antidepressant painstakingly slowly by such small reductions that the tapering program will take more than four months

Mild, Moderate, and Severe
Withdrawal Reactions

Antidepressant withdrawal reactions can be characterized as mild, moderate, or severe. This is a global, or overall, assessment based on the patient's worst symptoms and their effects on the patient's level of functioning. Some severe withdrawal symptoms have a greater impact on one's day-to-day life than others. Severe dizziness, for example, can have a pervasive effect on one's ability to function, making it difficult to drive or walk, to climb stairs, to lift objects or utensils, or even to turn one's head in conversation. Table 3.3 summarizes the criteria for differentiating mild, moderate, and severe withdrawal reactions.

Mild withdrawal symptoms are noticeable, but are not terribly uncomfortable and do not affect the patient's ability to function. Moderate withdrawal symptoms are more uncomfortable and, as they worsen in intensity, can become annoying or irritating. In addition, a key difference separating mild withdrawal symptoms from moderate ones is that moderate withdrawal symptoms affect one's ability to think clearly and/or to function normally. This may range from a modest interference in carrying out normal activities—such as the need to "take it a little easy"—to more significant interference—such as trouble concentrating that makes it difficult to function normally at work.

Severe withdrawal symptoms include any serious or alarming symptoms, including suicidal thoughts, suicidal behavior, harm to oneself or to others, hallucinations, or manic-like reactions. These severe symptoms are discussed in greater detail in the next chapter. Severe withdrawal symptoms also include any debilitating symptoms, such as incapacitating dizziness that requires one to lie or sit still for periods of time. Withdrawal symptoms are severe whenever they force patients to put the antidepressant dose back up or restart the drug if it had been stopped altogether. They are also severe if they force the patient to taper the drug painstakingly slowly by such small reductions that the tapering program will take more than four months.

4

How Changing the Dose of Antidepressants Up or Down May Make Patients Suicidal

Karen: A Case of Antidepressant Toxicity

Karen was weaving through the back streets of San Francisco, driving home from work at the end of the day, when she felt a knife-like pain in her abdomen. The pain was so severe Karen had to pull over to the side of the road. "Not again," Karen winced, recognizing the pain as a burst ovarian cyst. This was the third time in six months that she had had a cyst burst, causing severe pain. Karen endured waves of pain for about thirty minutes before she felt able to drive again. "I'd better get to the gynecologist again," she thought as the pain eased enough for her to pull back out into the traffic and make her way home.

In her late twenties, Karen had been living and working in San Francisco for five years. Originally from suburban Boston, she had gone to Pomona College in California and "migrated" up to San Francisco after graduating. A biology major, Karen landed a job as a paralegal in a law firm specializing in filing patents for biotechnology companies. Karen enjoyed the work so much that she was studying for the Law School Admission Test, or LSAT, and planning on applying to law school. She was in a warm, supportive relationship of three years with her boyfriend Alex. "Life was good," says Karen, looking back wistfully. "I was actively engaged in my work and a wonderful relationship. I was planning on going to law school. I was in great shape. I jogged five miles every other day. Little did I know what was about to befall me."

To stop the ovarian cyst pain, Karen's gynecologist recommended she go on the birth control pill. Ovarian cysts burst because they grow too large. The pill is thought to suppress ovarian cyst formation because of the hormonal regulation it introduces. However, Karen was reluctant because she had tried the pill once before and become very emotional and mildly depressed, a well-known side effect of oral contraceptives. This is not true clinical depression but rather a drug-induced side effect that looks like depression.[1] Karen's gynecologist assured her that the pill had changed considerably in the years since she had first taken it. It would likely not affect her in the same way, and was the best option for controlling the severe pain she was experiencing.

Karen agreed and began taking the pill, but this time it made her much more depressed. Within two weeks of starting the drug, Karen was having trouble getting out of bed and was crying much of the time. Her gynecologist immediately stopped the pill and referred her to a psychiatrist. Although the psychiatrist recognized that the birth control pill had caused Karen's depressive symptoms, instead of waiting for them to pass, he suggested the antidepressant Paxil. Karen reluctantly agreed, trusting the psychiatrist's judgment.

After starting Paxil, Karen gradually developed a number of side effects: nausea, vomiting, insomnia, dizziness, restlessness, and a rash. The rash covered her neck, back, and legs and lasted the entire time Karen was on the drug. The dizziness made her feel "wobbly," and was most pronounced whenever she changed position: rising up or sitting down. The restlessness made it difficult for Karen to lie or sit still. She was constantly fidgeting and shifting her posture. All her life, Karen had been a good sleeper. But, on Paxil, she could get only two hours of sleep a night. Night after night she lay awake for five and six hours at a time staring at the ceiling, tossing and turning in bed. "The insomnia really wore me down," says Karen. "I started feeling edgy and having difficulty concentrating during the day. I startled easily. Background noise in restaurants and other public places suddenly became menacing."

Within weeks of starting Paxil, Karen experienced the first panic attack in her life. She was out to dinner with friends at a busy, congested restaurant when she had a full-blown panic attack. Karen's legs began shaking as her heart started pounding in her chest. She rapidly became flushed, sweaty, and short of breath. "I was terrified," says Karen. "I didn't know what was happening to me." Karen had to cut the evening short. One of her friends left the dinner with her to take her home. Thereafter, she began having panic attacks on a regular basis.

In addition to the panic attacks, Karen began having fainting spells. Sometimes the fainting would occur after a panic attack. At other times, Karen fainted without first having had a panic attack. The first time she fainted, Karen's boyfriend, Alex, heard a thud in the next room, rushed in, and found her lying on the floor. Karen had no memory of what had happened. She later found out her blood pressure was dropping to dangerously low levels during the fainting spells.

Karen's psychiatrist did not recognize the panic attacks as side effects of the Paxil. Instead, he diagnosed her with panic disorder, started her on a Valium-type antianxiety agent, and increased her Paxil dose. He reassured her the Paxil was just not working yet but soon would. In addition, Karen began seeing a therapist who specialized in anxiety disorders.

About every two weeks, Karen's Paxil dose was rapidly increased—from 10 to 20 to 30 to 40 milligrams a day. Each time the dose was increased, Karen's symptoms became worse. She went months with no more than three hours of sleep at a time. What little sleep she got was disturbed by haunting, violent dreams. She became paranoid in public places, convinced that strangers had weapons and were hunting her down. She was afraid to leave her house. Her boyfriend and friends feared leaving her alone because of the danger posed by the fainting spells. "I couldn't drive a car because of the fainting," says Karen. "I had to quit my job. My life became more and more constricted as I focused what little energy I had on coping with my 'illness.' " Karen lived off savings and support from her family, who were back in Boston and increasingly concerned about her condition. Karen was also gaining significant weight on the drugs. She eventually gained seventy pounds.

Karen had started Paxil in September. By late December, her psychiatrist decided the Paxil was not working and switched her to Celexa. He was still operating on the premise that her symptoms were due to her worsening psychiatric condition rather than the drugs. During the winter, Karen's Paxil dose was stepped down from 40 to 20 to 10 to 0 milligrams a day, while her Celexa dose was increased from 10 to 20 to 40 to 60 to 80 milligrams a day, twice the maximum dose recommended by the FDA.[2] The insomnia, panic attacks, rash, nausea, vomiting, fainting spells, nightmares, and paranoia worsened each time the Celexa dose was increased.

On New Year's Eve, Karen became suicidal for the first time. "I pushed myself through the Christmas holiday but then I couldn't face the New Year. I just couldn't go on. I felt hopeless and helpless. I was suicidal for a week. It's a miracle I didn't kill myself. Alex saved my life keeping vigil over me."

"The whole winter, spring, and summer were a nightmare, as the drug side effects just got worse and worse," says Alex. "Of course we didn't know it was the drugs at the time. The psychiatrist kept saying, 'The next time we go up on the dose the Celexa will kick in and you'll feel back to normal again. You'll see. It's like a light bulb turns on and you feel fine again. Just hang in there.' We hung in there but it never happened. Karen just got worse and worse."

Karen's grandmother died in January, which distracted her from her suicidality. Karen was too ill to travel to the funeral. But her grandmother's death made her feel like she "finally had something to feel sad about that made sense."

Unfortunately, Karen's condition continued to deteriorate: She began having hallucinations of her grandmother's coffin. But as she approached the coffin, Karen would see her mother's dead body instead and become terrified. Karen repeatedly hallucinated a dog attacking and biting her in her apartment. She also heard voices (auditory hallucinations) telling her to harm herself. Haunted by the vivid hallucinations, now even Karen's home seemed to be unsafe. Karen's psychiatrist prescribed an antipsychotic that helped reduce the hallucinations. Karen was now taking eight to ten pills a day, a "cocktail" of antidepressants, Valium-type antianxiety agents, and antipsychotics.

"It's hard to imagine the transformation in Karen," says one of her closest friends, Melanie. "She went from this strong, healthy, outgoing person to an anxious, frightened, child-like shadow of herself. After I visited her sometimes I'd leave a wreck it was so awful watching what was happening to her."

In the early spring, Karen had her first episode of self-harm. "I was in the kitchen washing dishes and the next thing I knew I was lying on the floor, having cut and scratched myself with a kitchen knife. I have no memory of doing it. I washed my legs off. None of the cuts needed stitches. This happened several more times over the course of months."

In May, Karen began self-medicating with alcohol. In June, she added cocaine. She had no prior history of abusing drugs or alcohol. "They actually worked better for me than the prescription drugs, which I continued to take," says Karen. "I was horrified by what I was doing, but I was desperate." Feeling a little better, by the spring Karen was able to go back to work part-time. She also had laparoscopic surgery for the ovarian cysts, the original problem for which she had sought help.

Unfortunately, Karen was quickly fired from her job, in part because she was not functioning well. "Getting fired was a real blow," says Karen. "I've always been a superfunctional person, the last person who would get fired from a job." Thereafter, she worked sporadically at part-time jobs. In July, Karen's psychiatrist added Wellbutrin to the Celexa. Karen took the Wellbutrin only briefly because on it she felt worse, even more anxious and panicky.

Over the summer, Karen's friends and family confronted her about her drinking and cocaine use. Karen stopped the cocaine first. By September, she had stopped the alcohol too, and began going regularly to Alcoholics Anonymous. Unfortunately, when she stopped self-medicating Karen felt worse again: "I had been using the alcohol to calm myself down. Without it I became agitated again. Sobriety brought my illness back full force."

By now, Karen had been on antidepressants for a year. Her psychiatrist suggested switching from Celexa to Lexapro, saying that it might cause fewer side effects. Karen made the change in October. Within a week of starting Lexapro, she began having debilitating headaches. Karen asked her psychiatrist if the Lexapro could cause headaches and he said no, he had never heard of that. One night the headaches were so severe that Karen became suicidal and asked her upstairs neighbor to take her to the emergency room. "They gave me a CAT scan, tried to knock me out with intravenous pain medication, and sent me home. But the next day the headaches were worse. I knew I wouldn't be safe in my apartment, so I checked myself into a psychiatric ward. I spent the weekend in the hospital more frightened than ever. Insurance issues forced me to leave the hospital. Instead of going to another hospital in the Bay area, my family wanted me to fly home to Boston. I boarded a plane for Boston in early November, accompanied by my friend Melanie, having no idea that the hardest part was yet to come."

Even before Karen arrived home, her family began assembling a team to treat her. Karen's father is a doctor at a Harvard hospital. Her mother has a master's in public health and is a hospital administrator. So her family is well connected to the medical community. Karen grew up in Newton, a suburb of Boston. She has one younger sister.

Karen's mother, Claire, contacted a psychotherapist who had seen Karen briefly for a few sessions when she was in college. At the time Karen was dealing with normal developmental issues of college students, involving career choices and relationships. Together, Claire and the psychotherapist found a psychiatrist, a family doctor, and an acupuncturist to evaluate her. As Claire began to realize how sick Karen was, how much care she was going to require at home, and how much coordination her treatment would need, she decided to take a family medical leave of absence from her job to devote herself full time to seeing her daughter restored to health. "The Karen I knew was gone," says Claire. "She had been psychotic, paranoid, and suicidal. She still had the panic attacks, insomnia, rashes, fainting spells, and violent nightmares. She'd gained seventy pounds. She'd been like this for over a year. We knew she had been self-medicating with cocaine and alcohol for a brief part of that time. Karen had no confidence left. She couldn't advocate for herself. She couldn't keep track of her appointments because she was having trouble with her memory, with concentrating and thinking straight. I quickly realized how enormous my role would be."

Says Karen: "The severity of my symptoms and the length of time they had persisted left me completely devoid of the ability to advocate for myself. The health care system and medications had conspired together to separate me from me. My once strong internal compass had disappeared. I was unable to tell my own story and to relay my true feelings. I had lost access to a patient's most valuable resource—myself. My mom stepped in and became my advocate and my voice."

Even before Karen arrived home, the psychotherapist raised the possibility that she was suffering from antidepressant toxicity given the relentless worsening of her condition as her dose was steadily increased. "I was shocked," says Karen. "I thought the medication was supposed to be helping. It was such an alien idea."

"We were all shocked," says Claire, "but we wanted to keep an open mind to any possibility."

The day after Karen arrived in Boston, she met with a psychiatrist on the staff of Massachusetts General Hospital. The psychiatrist offered an alternative explanation for Karen's deterioration: "People who have trouble with antidepressants are often bipolar and don't know it," she said. "The antidepressant triggers mania or hypomania." Mania is also known as manic depressive illness, or bipolar disorder, for the two poles of mania and depression. Hypomania is a milder version of mania and is also known as Bipolar II. The psychiatrist suggested that Karen was Bipolar II. This diagnosis would mean more rather than less medication. The psychiatrist was opposed to taking Karen off her antidepressant. Reluctantly, she did agree to switch Karen's antidepressant back to Celexa from the Lexapro because friends of Karen's family had discovered on the Internet that Lexapro caused severe headaches in other patients.

Two days after Karen stopped the Lexapro, the headaches went away. She still had all the other symptoms, but the headaches, which began only when she started the Lexapro, were gone once she stopped it. The severe headaches had been the straw that broke the camel's back. They had driven Karen to the emergency room, to checking into a psychiatric ward, and ultimately to coming home. The headaches' disappearing so quickly after she stopped the Lexapro lent credence to the idea that she was suffering from antidepressant toxicity.

"Why don't doctors know Lexapro can cause severe headaches?" asked Karen. "I've since learned that doctors rely on pharmaceutical company sales reps for most of their information on drugs, so maybe that's the explanation. But here we were talking to top specialists in the country while having to go to the Internet for the real information."

Next, Karen met with the psychotherapist and the acupuncturist. These two meetings were the turning point in Karen's mind: "They each met with me for one to two hours to take detailed, thorough histories. They were the first clinicians all year to treat me like I was a valuable resource in diagnosing my condition and leading the charge on my road to wellness."

The psychotherapist had known Karen briefly in college. "I knew Karen before all this happened to her," says the therapist. "I was skeptical that in the absence of prexisting issues with mood that the person I had seen could have developed the symptoms Karen was suffering from. That's why I raised the possibility of antidepressant toxicity." Karen's therapist thought of antidepressant toxicity because she had read my earlier book, *Prozac Backlash*, which describes the side effects of antidepressants in detail.[3] "Karen had been started on an antidepressant too quickly," the therapist points out, "instead of waiting for the depression caused by the birth control pill to pass once she was off the pill. Then the dose was raised quickly and one antidepressant was added on top of another. All the terrible symptoms coincided with the drugs and with increasing the dose. My husband is a family doctor who prescribes antidepressants to patients, and he agreed it was a possibility. He's seen people have toxic reactions."

The acupuncturist worked closely with Karen throughout her treatment in Boston. Karen describes the acupuncture as a crucial part of her recovery. Says the acupuncturist of their first meeting: "I know Karen felt like she couldn't advocate for herself. She was totally bereft. But what I saw, even though she was debilitated, was this incredibly strong person, holding on for dear life trying to come back."

At this point, Karen had been on antidepressants for fourteen months. She had suffered nausea, vomiting, severe sleep deprivation, panic attacks, rashes, headaches, fainting spells, paranoia, hallucinations, cutting herself, and suicidal urges. Her relationship with her boyfriend, Alex, her career, and her entire life in San Francisco as she had known it had been casualties of her ordeal. Says the psychotherapist: "I saw Karen as heroic in the face of a body that was assaulting her."

The decision to taper Karen off Celexa was not an easy one. Karen's mother Claire and the psychotherapist talked to about a dozen psychiatrists who were unwilling to consider such a course of action. Over and over again they encountered the bipolar hypothesis. "It was maddening, especially given what we know now," says Claire. "How many people suffer antidepressant toxicity and are told it's bipolar disorder? Sure, the antipsychotic had helped with the hallucinations. Sure, the antianxiety agent [a Valium-type medication] was helping with the panic. Sure, antimanic drugs might have helped, too. But it was all the drugs. How many people are walking around overmedicated when the drugs are the real problem?"

Eventually, Claire found a psychiatrist willing to taper Karen off the Celexa even though he was not supportive or encouraging about the plan. "I appreciate his willingness to respect my wishes," says Karen, "even though he didn't buy the toxicity idea. I began tapering off the Celexa with incredible trepidation. I wasn't at all sure the drugs had caused my symptoms. It was such a paradigm shift. Little did I know the worst was yet to come."

Karen's new psychiatrist tapered her off the Celexa fairly steeply given the severity of the withdrawal symptoms she experienced. Over the course of just six and a half weeks her dose was reduced about every one to two weeks, from 80 milligrams a day to 60 to 40 to 20 to 10 to 5 to 0. Karen's medical withdrawal symptoms included severe dizziness ("I felt like I was falling, like I was in an elevator that went into free fall when I moved. Even if I just moved my eyes"); nausea and vomiting so severe it had to be treated with an antivomiting drug called compazine; flu-like aches and pains; severe, painful muscle spasms that sometimes produced involuntary movements; twitching all over her body including eye twitching; trembling ("I couldn't hold a pencil to write"); buzzing in her ears; electric shock–like sensations radiating down her back to the rest of her body that would lead to shaking for several minutes; and episodes Karen described as "brain freezes," painful shock-like sensation behind her eyes, accompanied by disorientation and brief amnesia without loss of consciousness.

A number of Karen's medical withdrawal symptoms raised concerns that she was having serious neurological events, including the "brain freezes" that led to brief amnesia and the shooting electric shock–like sensations that produced trembling and shaking so severe that Karen would have to lie down and looked like she was having convulsions. Says the family doctor who had become part of Karen's treating team: "She was getting worse and worse as she went down on the dose. We were all worried about her. We were concerned she might be having seizures or had a brain tumor. I ordered a whole battery of medical tests, including an MRI [a brain scan that looks for tumors] and an EEG [a brain wave that looks for evidence of seizures]. The MRI came back normal but the EEG was very abnormal."

When I spoke with the neurologist who did the EEG, he explained: "While Karen was on the table having the EEG, she had several episodes of the 'brain freezes' and electric shock–like sensations. The EEG showed high amplitude spike-and-slow-wave discharges, which can be seen in seizures. Based on the EEG, we felt a number of her symptoms were probably seizures. So we added an anticonvulsant to Karen's medications."

Still worse were Karen's psychiatric withdrawal symptoms: severe anxiety and insomnia ("Even worse than before I started to taper off the Celexa"); crying spells ("All the time."); confusion ("One day I stepped off the curb in front of an oncoming car I was so out of it. The car knocked me over but fortunately I wasn't seriously injured"); severe agitation and irritability; suicidal urges; and finally auditory hallucinations called "command hallucinations," voices telling Karen to kill herself and her parents.

The suicidal urges first appeared on day 2 after Karen reduced her Celexa dose from 60 to 40 milligrams a day. "I hadn't realized how bad the day was going to be and I'd gone to the gym in the morning thinking if I exercised a little that might make me feel better," says Karen. "Doing a Nautilus circuit, I had two brain freezes while on the machines. I was scared, and I left the gym. Driving home, I had this sudden, frightening thought: 'I should drive into that tree.' The urge came out of nowhere and was terrifying. Afterwards, I had more violent, scary thoughts. I became convinced my sister was dead." After this frightening episode, Karen did not feel safe driving; her family drove her everywhere.

But the worst withdrawal symptoms of all were the suicidal auditory hallucinations, which began three days later. "I heard two voices," says Karen. "One was the angry voice of a man demanding that I kill myself and my parents. I spent whole days and nights arguing with him. He kept insisting that I couldn't trust my parents or my doctors because they were killing me with these medications and I needed to kill them first. He made me so paranoid it became a real struggle. The other was a woman's voice cackling and murmuring in the background the whole time I was arguing with the man's voice."

The auditory hallucinations became so loud and intense in the last two weeks of the taper that Karen, her family, and her doctors did not feel she was safe at home. "The last night I was home," says Karen, "the voices kept insisting I had to kill my mother. I was up all night, terrified. I wanted to wake my father and tell him what was happening. But the voice kept insisting I couldn't tell my father either. In the morning I told my parents what had happened. That's when everyone decided this was no longer safe and I needed to be admitted to the hospital." Karen was admitted to a Harvard hospital for the end of the taper. There she was watched vigilantly, twenty-four hours a day.

While in the hospital, Karen made the last two dosage reductions and stopped the Celexa altogether. Despite high doses of antipsychotic medication, Karen continued to hear the voices the entire twelve days she was in the hospital. Indeed, she was still hearing them when she was discharged six days after her last Celexa dose. But the voices were much lower in volume and intensity, so everyone on her treatment team felt it was safe to send Karen home. Nine days after stopping Celexa, the voices went away completely and have not returned. Within a month, almost all of Karen's symptoms disappeared, including the suicidal thoughts, nightmares, dizziness, fainting spells, panic attacks, paranoia, rashes, nausea, vomiting, buzzing in her ears, tingling sensations, waves of electric shock–like sensations, and "brain freezes." The residual symptoms that took many months to slowly improve were the insomnia and the painful muscle cramping. Karen also had erratic mood swings in the first few months off the drugs. As her symptoms improved, Karen weaned off all the other medications, including the sleeping pills, Valium-type anti-anxiety agents, antipsychotics, and anticonvulsant. Karen lived with her family for three more months before she felt strong enough to go back to San Francisco to try to reclaim her life.

"My family was scared about my going back so soon," says Karen. "Everyone wanted me to stay in Boston longer. But I felt ripped out of my life. Back in San Francisco, it felt strange trying to reclaim who I was. Some people treated me like 'We had such a hard time believing you were a crazy woman—now you're telling us you're not?' But most people have been terrific. I even went back to my old job. I couldn't believe they were willing to give me another chance. I can remember the first time I had to write up a long legal brief. I was wondering, 'Can I do this?' I knew they were wondering the same thing. I did fine."

Karen's relationship with her boyfriend, Alex, did not survive the ordeal. "He was so good for so long, but eventually it took its toll that I was so crazed on the drugs. We're back to being good friends. He's been very supportive." Still on hold are the plans Karen had to take the LSAT and apply to law school. "It may be too late for that," she says wistfully. "But maybe not, I'm just taking it a step at a time." Karen is back to exercising regularly and jogs five days a week, about five miles each time. She's lost some, but not all, of the seventy pounds she gained on the drugs.

I first met Karen when I was invited by her treatment team to attend a grand rounds, a medical case conference sponsored jointly by the department of medicine and the department of psychiatry at the Harvard hospital where she was treated. Karen returned from the West Coast to attend the conference, which was held after she had been off Celexa for a year. Addressing the large audience in the hospital's auditorium, Karen described her harrowing ordeal with extraordinary poise and equanimity. In addition to Karen, the audience heard presentations by Karen's mother, psychotherapist, acupuncturist, family doctor, neurologist, and the head of inpatient psychiatry at the hospital. Karen's extraordinary case is carefully documented in the medical records of the many clinicians who treated her, starting with her psychiatrist and gynecologist in San Francisco.

"Looking back on it," says Karen, "I think: Why wasn't the rash an early sign that I was having an allergic reaction to the antidepressants?

Under ordinary circumstances, I never would have put up with the rash. But the panic attacks, sleep deprivation, and severe psychiatric symptoms all happened so fast that they became the focus. The rash seemed the least of my problems."

"There's been a lot of attention to children having bad reactions to antidepressants," says Karen's mother, Claire. "I think that's because children are so defenseless and dependent on adults to advocate for them. But as Karen's case illustrates, adults suffering from antidepressant toxicity can become defenseless and no longer able to advocate for themselves, too. Some adults may be more vulnerable than children because they don't have parents or other family members keeping a close eye on them. The doctors who treat them don't know them as well as family and don't recognize the dramatic changes brought about by the drugs. Instead, they interpret it as mental illness."

Says Karen's psychotherapist, reflecting on her ordeal: "This happened because the psychiatrist in California was too quick to prescribe antidepressants and then never stopped to consider that the drugs might be the problem."

"I'm still angry over how many times psychiatrists suggested I was bipolar," says Karen. "Halfway through the taper off Celexa, my psychiatrist in Boston brought it up again. 'Maybe all of this is because you're bipolar,' he said. It felt like a trick, a way of blaming me instead of the drugs. I had no history of ever being manic. I had no history of ever being depressed, except as a drug-induced side effect of birth control pills. I had no history of panic attacks, psychosis, or being suicidal. It was all the drugs!"

The failure of Karen's psychiatrist in San Francisco to consider that the drugs might be the problem is a disturbing phenomenon. Prior to 2004, doctors were almost never sued over toxic reactions to antidepressants, even when patients committed suicide. This is because bereaved families have considered pharmaceutical companies to be the culprits. The pharmaceutical industry's failure to warn about the side effects even afforded doctors some protection. But the FDA's 2004 warnings shift more of the responsibility to doctors. Indeed, with lawsuits against pharmaceutical companies burgeoning, the industry may have quietly supported the warnings because they shift liability onto doctors. Doctors can no longer afford to be ill-informed about antidepressant-induced suicidality, even if the pharmaceutical industry and the FDA make only minimal efforts to educate them about it.

The March 2004 FDA warning states that patients can be particularly vulnerable "at the beginning of therapy or when the dose either increases or decreases," that is, whenever the dose *changes*.[4] The warning cites a range of antidepressant side effects, many illustrated by Karen's case, that can contribute to patients becoming suicidal or more dangerously suicidal, including "anxiety, agitation, panic attacks, insomnia, irritability, hostility, akathisia (severe restlessness), hypomania, and mania." These side effects are generally known as "paradoxical" side effects since they cause a worsening of the patient's condition that may include worsening of preexisting suicidality or the development of new suicidal thoughts and behavior.[5]

The FDA warnings apply to all eleven of the antidepressants we have been discussing: Paxil, Zoloft, Celexa, Lexapro, Luvox, Prozac, Effexor, Cymbalta, Serzone, Remeron, and Wellbutrin. More research is needed to clarify how antidepressants can contribute to suicidality. Questions that need to be answered include: Are some of today's antidepressants more likely than others to cause suicide and violence?[6] What percentage of patients become suicidal when their antidepressant dose changes? Of the patients who become suicidal, what percentage suffer from each of the antidepressant side effects associated with suicidality—that is, insomnia, anxiety, panic attacks, akathisia (drug-induced agitation), irritability, hostility, impulsivity (disinhibition), manic-like reactions, paranoid reactions, and psychotic reactions? What are the similarities and differences between antidepressant-induced suicidality when patients start the drugs and increase the dose versus when they decrease the dose in midtreatment or when tapering off the drugs?

Antidepressant-induced suicide and violence came to the attention of the media, the public, the medical profession, and the FDA in the early 1990s, shortly after Prozac, the first of today's antidepressants, was introduced. At the time Prozac was associated with a number of dramatic suicides and murder-suicides.[7] In addition to sensational media reports, psychiatrists published numerous reports and small-scale studies of antidepressant-induced suicidality in medical journals.[8] Because of public and professional concern, the FDA and Eli Lilly, Prozac's manufacturer, agreed to a large-scale, systematic study of the phenomenon.[9] Lilly worked with expert consultants to develop the protocols for the study. As part of the effort, Lilly developed more sensitive rating scales for assessing suicidality in antidepressant studies.[10] At the time, the rest of today's antidepressants were at various stages of being studied to gain

FDA approval. Lilly could have provided the more sensitive rating scales for assessing suicidality to other pharmaceutical companies with new antidepressants in the pipeline to use in their studies. Unfortunately, once the media attention to the problem in the early 1990s died down, the issue was swept under the carpet. Lilly never did the study of antidepressant-induced suicidality, which might have saved countless lives in the past decade. The FDA failed to see that the study was done. And the FDA did not require pharmaceutical companies developing the many other new antidepressants that followed Prozac to use the more sensitive scales for assessing antidepressant-induced suicidality in their studies of the drugs.

Given the pharmaceutical industry's resistance to this much-needed research, it is not likely to be done for years. In the meantime, doctors, patients, and their families need to be vigilant for paradoxical worsening of a patient's condition, especially when the dose of an antidepressant changes. Unfortunately, doctors like Karen's, who are unaware of antidepressant-induced suicidality, can stare the side effect in the face and not recognize it because they mistake it for a worsening of the patient's underlying psychiatric condition. Over and over again in some of the most tragic cases, doctors who did not recognize the side effect have relentlessly increased the dose as the patient got worse and worse.

Table 4.1 lists the antidepressant side effects that may make patients suicidal. The list is based on the FDA warnings, warnings in other countries (including Britain and Canada), the warnings that have been issued by pharmaceutical companies in response to these regulatory actions, and the published reports of experts on this phenomenon.[11] Note that these are side effects that can occur in anyone put on the drugs, not just depressed patients. Many of the patients who have become suicidal on antidepressants were not depressed or suicidal before going on the drugs. Instead, they were put on the drugs for conditions such as headaches, back pain, or chronic fatigue syndrome. Because more research is needed in this critical area, the list in Table 4.1 and the discussion that follows are not meant to be exhaustive or definitive. Instead, the goal is to heighten awareness among doctors, patients, and families of the potential danger posed by antidepressants while we all await additional research that will provide more definitive information.

Table 4.1 ANTIDEPRESSANT SIDE EFFECTS
THAT MAY MAKE PATIENTS SUICIDAL

Insomnia

Anxiety/panic attacks

Akathisia (drug-induced agitation)

Irritability/hostility/impulsivity (disinhibition)

Mania-like reactions

Paranoid reactions

Psychotic reactions

Insomnia

Insomnia is perhaps the easiest side effect of antidepressants for nonprofessionals to understand heightening the risk of suicide. Have you ever been sleepless for nights on end? Have you gotten two or three hours of fitful sleep a night and otherwise tossed and turned in bed, staring at the ceiling, ruminating about your worries, desperate for the peace a good night's sleep would offer? Severe sleep deprivation impairs people's judgment and makes them edgy and more impulsive. Chronic sleep deprivation can lead to despair, a fear on the patient's part that if she cannot sleep, she will eventually lose her mind.[12] Under these circumstances, patients are more vulnerable to acting on suicidal thoughts or urges.

Psychiatrists have long recognized that insomnia heightens the risk of suicide. Repeated studies have examined the link between them.[13] Experts refer to insomnia as a "modifiable suicide risk factor," because it can be identified and potentially treated.[14] Depending on its severity, insomnia is treated by a variety of means, including better sleep hygiene, exercise, herbal sleep remedies, and prescription sleeping pills.

Antidepressant-induced insomnia can be even more pernicious than insomnia that is not drug-induced. This is especially true when the doctor and patient are not aware of the real cause of the problem. Under these circumstances, efforts to treat the insomnia are more likely to fail because the underlying problem is not addressed. Indeed, in a vicious cycle, at the same time that the patient is put on a sleeping pill, the dose of the antidepressant is likely to be increased in an effort to "treat" the patient's worsening "illness." This is akin to putting one foot on the brake and simultaneously putting the other on the gas pedal.

Doctors and patients need to be aware that many of today's antidepressants can cause insomnia as a side effect. The dose of the antidepressant may need to be lowered. Sometimes the insomnia clears on the lower dose as the patient adjusts to the medication and then one can try going back up more slowly on the dose. In other instances, one needs to taper off the antidepressant. Sometimes switching to a more sedating antidepressant works.

Anxiety and Panic Attacks

Experts also refer to anxiety and panic attacks as "modifiable suicide risk factors," since they are potentially treatable.[15] The term "anxiety" refers to the psychological state of being anxious, tense, fearful, or worried. The term "panic attack" refers to the physical symptoms that can accompany severe anxiety: racing heart, shortness of breath, chest pain, feeling faint, hot flashes, sweating, trembling, tingling sensations, and a fear that one is losing one's mind or dying.[16] Most people think of depressed patients as the most likely to become suicidal. In fact, studies have shown that anxious patients are as likely as depressed patients to become suicidal.[17] The combination of depression and anxiety can be particularly deadly. Like insomnia, anxiety can impair people's judgment and make them frightened, panicky, impulsive, and at greater risk of suicide.

Most doctors are familiar with today's antidepressants making patients anxious or panicky. Patients starting antidepressants or increasing the dose often feel "caffeinated," to the point of becoming jittery. This is because today's antidepressants can be overstimulating for some patients. Patients sometimes have to cut back on their caffeine intake while adjusting to antidepressants. Other patients simply cannot tolerate the drugs because they make them so anxious. A particularly dangerous scenario is when antidepressants make patients anxious on top of being depressed, heightening the risk of their becoming suicidal. When patients decrease the dose or taper off antidepressants, anxiety is one of the most common psychiatric withdrawal symptoms.

Some of today's antidepressants, like Zoloft, are approved by the

FDA to treat panic disorder. However, if one looks carefully at the prescribing guidelines for Zoloft, the recommended starting dose for panic disorder is half the recommended starting dose for depression.[18] This is because antidepressants can make anxiety worse. The fact that antidepressants can be used to treat anxiety in some patients while the drugs cause anxiety in others is just part of the paradoxical reactions they can cause in different patients.

Anxiety that is not drug-induced can be treated by a variety of means, including cognitive-behavioral treatment, psychotherapy, exercise, herbal antianxiety agents, and prescription antianxiety (usually Valium-type) drugs. Antidepressant-induced anxiety is important to recognize as such, because it is too acute and too physiological to treat with cognitive-behavioral therapy or psychotherapy. Instead, depending on the severity of the anxiety, one needs to lower the dose, stop the drug, add antianxiety agents, and/or switch to a more sedating antidepressant.

Akathisia (Drug-induced Agitation)

Of the paradoxical, overstimulating side effects of antidepressants, perhaps the least well-known to family doctors is akathisia, a severe form of drug-induced agitation that has long been linked to suicide and violence.[19] Akathisia is a well established side effect of selective serotonin reuptake inhibitor antidepressants (SSRIs).[20] All of the manufacturers of SSRIs list akathisia as a side effect of the drugs.[21] Because of the reports of SSRI-induced akathisia published in medical journals, the American Psychiatric Association's *Diagnostic and Statistical Manual of Mental Disorders (DSM)*, the profession's official compendium of medical information, states: "Serotonin-specific reuptake inhibitor antidepressant medication may produce akathisia."[22] Moreover, the *DSM* spells out the connection between this side effect and suicide and violence: "The subjective distress resulting from akathisia is significant. . . . Akathisia may be associated with dysphoria [distress], irritability, *aggression, or suicide attempts* [emphasis added]." Other authoritative textbooks also describe antidepressant-induced akathisia.[23] Unfortunately, most primary care doctors, who write the vast majority of prescriptions for antidepressants, are unaware the drugs can cause akathisia and that akathisia may in turn cause suicide and violence. Even many psychiatrists are unaware of this crucial link between antidepressants, suicide, and violence.

Akathisia has two sides, or faces: outer, objective restlessness and inner, subjective agitation.[24] The outer, visible restlessness caused by akathisia particularly affects the legs and may be mild, moderate, or severe. In mild cases, patients find it difficult to sit or stand comfortably. They may adjust their posture frequently, shifting their weight from one foot to the other while standing, or crossing and uncrossing their legs while sitting. In moderate cases, patients are more visibly jittery and fidgety, tapping their feet on the floor or pacing. In severe cases, patients are visibly agitated, find it difficult to sit still, and are driven to pace back and forth.

The inner, subjective agitation of akathisia is, in fact, its more dangerous side. This drug-induced state can include anxiety, tension, irritability, hostility, paranoia, rage reactions, and violence. Akathisia has been described in medical journals as causing "abject terror" in patients.[25] Akathisia is unlike anything the patient has ever experienced before. Patients report: "I feel like I'm going to explode, like the molecules inside my body are all sped up, bursting against my skin." "I feel like my bones are tuning forks rattling in my body." "I feel like I'm living twenty-four hours a day with the sensation of nails scratching up and down a blackboard." "I feel like I have caffeine running in my veins." "I feel like jumping out of my skin."

Writing in medical journals, experts describe akathisia as "more difficult to endure than any of the symptoms for which they [patients] had been originally treated."[26] The abnormal bodily sensations and anxiety can make it difficult for patients to think clearly, leaving them with feelings of confusion and unreality. Indeed, as part of akathisia patients may experience depersonalization, an "out-of-body experience" in which they feel outside themselves, observing themselves, horrified by their suicidal or violent behavior, but unable to stop themselves. Experts refer to the effects of akathisia as a form of "behavioral toxicity" of antidepressants.[27]

Akathisia can be extremely dangerous, especially in patients who have not been warned about the side effect and mistake it for a worsening of their psychiatric condition. Akathisia can trigger panic reactions in patients, increase paranoia, and drive patients to suicide and violence.[28] Suicidal impulses can arise because of an obsessive preoccupation with suicide induced by akathisia. Some patients report that they become suicidal because death offers a welcome relief from the otherwise inescapable physical and psychological torment of akathisia.[29] Patients describe the suicidal urges as alien, intrusive, and completely out of character. Violent attacks or homicides can arise because of heightened paranoia, irritability, and rage reactions.[30] The suicidal and homicidal impulses are closely related manifestations of the same underlying agitation, impulsivity, and disinhibition caused by akathisia.

Typically, the suicidality of akathisia is distinctly different from the suicidality of depression. Patients who become suicidal as a result of akathisia are preoccupied with escaping the behavioral toxicity, anxiety, irritability, and abject terror of the physical and psychological state of akathisia. This involves a marked deterioration of the patient's condition that typically coincides with starting the drug or changing the dose. This is very different from the suicidality typically seen with depression. Depressed patients are preoccupied with guilt, self-loathing, and hopelessness. The guilt, self-loathing, and hopelessness are what they seek to escape by suicide. Depressed patients can be suicidal but are usually not homicidal in the way that patients with antidepressant-induced akathisia can be. In women in particular, antidepressant-induced suicidality is often much more violent than the suicidality seen in depression. Depressed women typically attempt suicide by overdosing rather than more violent means. But with antidepressant-induced suicidality, women typically attempt or commit suicide by unusually violent means: mutilating themselves with knives, hanging themselves, shooting themselves, or jumping off buildings. Says Harvard Medical School psychiatrist Dr. Jonathan Cole, one of the country's leading experts on psychiatric drugs: "The real suicidal drive caused by an SSRI often stands out from the patient's long-standing depression like pneumonia in a patient with a long history of dust allergies. If some cases stand out strikingly, there are logically others where the adverse effect is more subtle."[31] To further differentiate antidepressant-induced suicidality from the suicide of depression, one can stop the drug or prescribe a second drug that counteracts akathisia (see discussion of the treatment of akathisia below). If the akathisia and suicidality disappear, this helps to establish that they were drug-induced rather than caused by the patient's depression.

Patients vary widely in their vulnerability to developing akathisia. Not all patients who develop akathisia will become suicidal. Rather, a subset of patients with akathisia is driven to suicidal or violent behavior. In some antidepressant-induced suicides, autopsy studies have found the patients had low levels of the liver enzymes that metabolize and inactivate antidepressants. Because these patients were "poor metabolizers," they had abnormally high levels of the antidepressants in their blood despite being on recommended doses.

Akathisia is treated by stopping the antidepressant or adding a second drug to counteract the side effect. The drugs used to counteract akathisia while remaining on an SSRI are propranolol (a beta-blocker often prescribed to treat stage fright) and Ativan (a Valium-type antianxiety agent).[32] My preference is to stop the drug since this is such a dangerous side effect. Unfortunately, doctors who are unaware of antidepressant-induced suicidality typically do the opposite: they raise the dose because they mistake the drug-induced suicidality for a worsening of the patient's underlying psychiatric condition. But, in a vicious cycle, raising the dose worsens the problem. If one stops the drug and the patient still needs an antidepressant, after the patient has stabilized one can try an antidepressant in a different class, which may not cause the patient to have the same reaction.

Manic-like Reactions

Mania and hypomania are controversial side effects of antidepressants, as Karen's case illustrates. Mania is a severe psychiatric condition consisting of an elevated, or high, mood that can include grandiosity, rapid speech, racing thoughts, irritability, distractability, agitation, insomnia, reckless behavior (e.g., buying sprees or sexual indiscretions), delusions, and hallucinations. Hypomania is a milder version of mania. This relatively new psychiatric diagnosis became officially established only in the mid-1990s. At the time, mania was officially renamed Bipolar I so that hypomania could be named Bipolar II.

Antidepressants can certainly make patients look manic or hypomanic. But the American Psychiatric Association's *Diagnostic and Statistical Manual (DSM)* explicitly states that "manic-like [or hypomanic-like] episodes that are clearly caused by somatic antidepressant treatment (e.g. medication . . .) should not count toward a diagnosis of Bipolar I [or Bipolar II] Disorder," because these are drug-induced states.[33]

But pharmaceutical companies and psychiatrists who are zealous drug proponents have misled countless patients and doctors to believe that antidepressant-induced manic-like states indicate the patient has an underlying bipolar illness that was merely "brought out," or triggered, by the drug. The *DSM* also states clearly that "no laboratory findings [i.e. tests] that are diagnostic of a Manic Episode have been identified."[34] In other words, there is no blood test, X-ray, brain scan, or any other test to objectively, definitively diagnose someone with a bipolar disorder. Instead, bipolar disorder is a diagnosis made on the basis of the patient's behavior and mental state. If a patient who is not on any drugs becomes manic, then one can reasonably conclude that the patient has bipolar disorder. But, if the manic-like state is caused by an antidepressant, this is a drug-induced state, which, although it may mimic bipolar disorder, is not actually bipolar disorder, as explicitly stated by the *DSM*, psychiatry's official diagnostic manual. Yet, in contrast to the *DSM*, every manufacturer of the eleven antidepressants we have been discussing has a warning in their official information on the drugs that antidepressants can cause "activation of mania/hypomania."[35] For example, GlaxoSmithKline says in its official information on Wellbutrin: "Antidepressants can precipitate manic episodes in Bipolar Manic Depressive patients during the depressed phase of their illness and may activate latent psychosis in other susceptible patients."[36] In recent years, the pharmaceutical industry has inundated doctors with "educational" material on "bipolar depression," promoting the idea that depressed patients like Karen, who became anxious, agitated, and sleepless on antidepressants, are bipolar: Bipolar II if the patients "just" become anxious, agitated, and sleepless; Bipolar I if they become paranoid, reckless, or psychotic. Bipolar I or Bipolar II, it doesn't matter, the "treatment" is more drugs, powerful antimanic agents.

For decades, lithium was the psychiatric drug used to treat bipolar disorder. Lithium is a naturally occurring salt, not a patented drug, so there is little or no money to be made on it. About a decade ago, pharmaceutical companies began promoting lucrative, patented anticonvulsant drugs to replace lithium for bipolar disorder. While lithium has serious side effects, so do these drugs, which include Tegretol, Depakote, Neurontin, Lamictal, Topamax, and Trileptal. When they were first promoted for bipolar disorder, many of these anticonvulsants were not approved by the FDA for this condition. Some of them, like Neurontin, never received FDA approval for bipolar disorder. In fact, in the last decade, the pharmaceutical industry's aggressive promotion of these drugs has become a scandal. In May 2004, Pfizer paid a $430 million settlement to resolve criminal charges and civil liabilities following a Department of Justice investigation into accusations that Pfizer's Warner-Lambert division had illegally promoted Neurontin for bipolar disorder and other conditions. An unpublished study conducted at Harvard allegedly suppressed by the company showed that Neurontin was worse than placebo (dummy) pills for bipolar disorder.[37] Yet, according to David Franklin, a former company sales representative who was a whistleblower in the federal lawsuits, the company trained its salespeople to tell doctors that Neurontin was so effective for bipolar disorder that "90 percent of patients had 90 percent recovery 90 percent of the time."[38] According to prosecutors the company also provided kickbacks to doctors who prescribed Neurontin to large numbers of patients with bipolar disorder.[39] The kickbacks were expensive travel and entertainment, which the company reported as consulting or medical education. The aggressive marketing was so effective that, by 2003, 90 percent of prescriptions for Neurontin were written for conditions like bipolar disorder, for which the drug is not approved by the FDA.[40] By 2003, Pfizer's sales of Neurontin reached $2.7 billion annually.[41] Says David Franklin: "I thought I was being hired to answer doctors' questions in a fair and balanced way. My job was actually to pervert the medical process and provide absolutely false and fabricated information to the physician. After seven and a half years of this case, we realize the depth of control these companies have over our health care."[42]

Bipolar II became an official psychiatric diagnosis in the mid-1990s, at the same time that pharmaceutical companies began aggressively promoting anticonvulsant drugs for bipolar patients. Prior to the 1990s, patients were only labeled bipolar if they had severe, usually psychotic, manic episodes. All this changed with the introduction of Bipolar II, or mild mania, which suddenly cast the bipolar net over many more patients. In recent decades, the definitions of a host of psychiatric diagnoses (including depression, obsessive compulsive disorder (OCD), and social phobia) have been watered down in this way to capture many more patients. In each instance, the phenomenon has been part of a carefully orchestrated effort to promote new drugs for the condition. In the process, previously rare (OCD and social phobia) or nonexistent (Bipolar II) diagnoses have suddenly become epidemics. Critics describe the phenomenon as marketing diseases to market drugs.[43] Psychiatric diagnoses are subject to this kind of manipulation because there are no objective medical tests by which to diagnose any psychiatric condition. The subjectivity of psychiatric diagnoses makes them vulnerable to commercial exploitation. When people take so much cocaine that they have manic-like reactions and end up in an emergency room, they are diagnosed with cocaine toxicity. When people have manic-like reactions to steroids, they are diagnosed with steroid toxicity. Yet when people have the same type of reactions to antidepressants, they are misdiagnosed with so-called "underlying bipolar disorder." The practice protects antidepressants and promotes antimanic agents, which have become multibillion-dollar-a-year drugs.

The Bipolar II diagnosis not only makes it easier to diagnose people with the dread disorder, it also makes it easier to establish a "prior history" of the condition. I have consulted with students who were diagnosed bipolar because they were up all night writing a paper. I have consulted with writers, artists, and filmmakers who were diagnosed bipolar because they had energetic periods in which they felt passionate about their work, even if they were not productive.

Some psychiatrists argue that patients who become manic on antidepressants are more likely to become manic again at a later date. Even if such a patient goes on to become manic again, the initial manic response to an antidepressant is not in and of itself proof of an underlying bipolar disorder. This would merely be an hypothesis, since there is no objective medical test with which to diagnose bipolar disorder. An equally plausible hypothesis would be that the antidepressant toxicity had lasting effects that left the patient more vulnerable to manic-like episodes in the future. When one sees patients who endure what Karen went through on antidepressants, this becomes a reasonable hypothesis.

Patients with bona fide, prior existing bipolar disorders may be a special case. These are patients with clear-cut, severe manic episodes (e.g., manic psychoses requiring hospitalization) that occurred before the patients took any drugs that can cause manic-like states. Patients with pre-existing bipolar disorder should only be prescribed an antidepressant if absolutely necessary and with great caution. If the antidepressant causes a manic-like episode, it can be difficult to distinguish from the patient's underlying Bipolar I disorder. Still, by the strict definition of the American Psychiatric Association's *Diagnostic and Statistical Manual,* the antidepressant-induced episode does "not count toward a diagnosis" of a bipolar disorder. The patient only carries the bipolar diagnosis because of the previously existing manic episode when she was drug-free. Adhering to this strict definition is the only way to avoid the overdiagnosis of bipolar disorder and marketing of diseases to market drugs that we have seen in the last decade.

Irritability, Hostility, and Impulsivity (Disinhibition)

The pharmaceutical companies' official information on almost all of today's antidepressants list irritability, hostility, or aggressive reactions as side effects of the drugs.[44] A good example of hostile, aggressive behavior resulting from antidepressant withdrawal is John in Chapter 3, the Harvard undergraduate who impulsively stole another student's backpack and charge cards while in severe Paxil withdrawal.

Notice the overlap among the antidepressant side effects linked to suicide and violence: Anxiety can cause insomnia. Conversely, insomnia can make people anxious. Both anxiety and insomnia can be manifestations of akathisia or manic-like reactions. According to psychiatrist Peter Breggin, what one is looking at is a cluster of overstimulating side effects of antidepressants that can heighten the risk of suicide and violence.[45] Anxiety, insomnia, akathisia, and manic-like reactions all, in turn, can lead to irritability, hostility, and impulsivity. Disinhibition is the technical name for impulsivity; it refers to loss of the normal inhibitions to suicidal and aggressive acts.

Paranoid Reactions

The official information of most of today's antidepressants list paranoia or paranoid reactions as side effects of the drugs.[46] Moreover, paranoia can accompany severe insomnia, anxiety, akathisia, or manic-like reactions. Paranoia leaves people suspicious, isolated, edgy, and frightened. Severe or chronic paranoia can make people feel persecuted and despairing. Paranoia can reach delusional, psychotic proportions. All these aspects of paranoia can heighten the risk of suicide or violence.

Psychotic Reactions

Psychosis is the state of being out of touch with reality. Psychosis manifests itself as delusions or hallucinations. Delusions are beliefs that are untrue. In an antidepressant-induced paranoid psychosis, Karen believed that strangers were carrying weapons and hunting her down. Hallucinations can be visual or auditory. Karen hallucinated her grandmother's coffin with her mother's dead body in it. She also hallucinated a dog attacking and biting her. During Celexa withdrawal, Karen heard voices, command hallucinations, telling her to kill herself and her parents. Obviously, being out of touch with reality endangers patients and heightens the risk of suicide or violence.

Energizing Patients

Long before the introduction of today's popular antidepressants, psychiatrists recognized that earlier classes of antidepressants could heighten the risk of suicide, especially in the early weeks and months when patients were starting the drugs and increasing the dose.[47] Psychiatrists thought that antidepressants had an energizing, or stimulating, effect that kicked in before the antidepressant effect occurred. In this early window of vulnerability shortly after starting the drugs or increasing the dose, patients could still be depressed but have the energy to act on suicidal thoughts—energy that they lacked before going on the stimulating drugs. This so-called "reenergizing" effect of earlier antidepressants was poorly understood. Earlier classes of antidepressants can also cause the side effects described above to varying degrees, depending on the particular drug. In all likelihood, what psychiatrists had been looking at with older antidepressants was, in fact, these side effects, which were less well understood. Today, we are witnessing a refinement of these early, decades old observations that antidepressants can heighten the risk of suicide.

Warning Patients Before They Go on Antidepressants

Patients need to be warned about antidepressant-induced suicidality before they go on the drugs and reminded again when they taper off. The most dangerous scenario is when patients are not warned about this side effect. Under these circumstances, patients mistake the side effect for a worsening of their condition and think "The miracle cure that's helped millions of people is not working for me. I'm a hopeless case," putting them at even greater risk to harm themselves. When patients are warned, no matter how badly an antidepressant may make them feel, they can always retain the idea that "This may be the drug, not me" and seek immediate medical attention. Doctors also need to be well informed in order to accurately diagnose and treat antidepressant-induced suicidality.

Unfortunately, until recently, a paternalistic approach has prevailed: "Don't warn patients, you might scare them away from treatment." Such an authoritarian approach has no place in contemporary medicine. Nothing is more dangerous and frightening than developing this side effect when one has not been warned. I warn patients routinely and they are not frightened away from treatment.

Monitoring Patients Closely

Whenever patients start antidepressants, go up on the dose, lower the dose in mid-treatment, or taper off the drugs, they need to be monitored closely to ensure their safety. Patients need to be fully informed of all the side effects discussed in this chapter that can cause or exacerbate suicidality and violence so they can monitor themselves at home between appointments with their doctor. When the patients are children, the families need to be fully informed so they can monitor their children at home.

The new 2004 FDA warnings recommend that children starting antidepressants should be seen by their doctor "at least weekly face-to-face . . . during the first four weeks of treatment, then biweekly visits for the next four weeks, then at twelve weeks, and as clinically indicated beyond twelve weeks. Additional contact by telephone may be appropriate between face-to-face visits."[48] A similarly high standard of care should apply to adults, since, as Karen's case illustrates, adults can become as vulnerable as children when they deteriorate on antidepressants. Ideally, adults should be seen by their doctor at least weekly for the first two to three weeks on the drug, at least once a month for the second and third month, and as clinically indicated thereafter. The same guidelines apply whenever patients increase the dose of their antidepressant, since each increase runs the risk again of antidepressant-induced deterioration in the patient's condition. I have sometimes met daily with patients who developed antidepressant-induced suicidality while we waited for the suicidality to clear after stopping the drug. Hospitalization may even be necessary, although I have always been able to manage this side effect on an outpatient basis, probably because it was recognized early on, before the patient deteriorated to the degree Karen did.

When monitoring patients, special attention needs to be paid to any deterioration in the patient's condition. When patients develop any of the side effects described in this chapter, the side effects need to be treated promptly and effectively. Says the FDA: "Consideration should be given to changing the therapeutic regimen, including possibly discontinuing the [antidepressant] medication, in patients whose depression [or other condition] is persistently worse, or who are experiencing [newly] emergent [or worsening] suicidality."[49] The FDA describes the kinds of side effects discussed in this chapter as potential "precursors to worsening depression or suicidality, especially if these symptoms are severe, abrupt in onset, or were not part of the patient's presenting symptoms," i.e., original condition.[50]

While the FDA's recommendations for closely monitoring patients are welcome, unfortunately the agency lists the antidepressant side effects that may lead to suicidality only as "anxiety, agitation, panic attacks, insomnia, irritability, hostility (aggressiveness), impulsivity, akathisia (psychomotor restlessness), hypomania and mania" without providing more details on how they may cause or aggravate suicidality. The one exception, the one side effect the FDA provides a full paragraph on, is antidepressants allegedly triggering mania and hypomania. Here the FDA is following the pharmaceutical industry's push to emphasize this side effect. While focusing on this alleged side effect, the FDA failed to provide doctors and patients with any details on akathisia despite the extensive medical reports and research linking it to antidepressant-induced suicidality and violence.

Says the FDA of mania and hypomania: "A major depressive episode may be the initial presentation of bipolar disorder. It is generally *believed* (*though not established* in controlled trials) that treating such an episode with an antidepressant alone may increase the likelihood of precipitation of a mixed/manic episode in patients at risk for bipolar disorder. *Whether any of the symptoms described above [i.e., antidepressant side effects like those described in this chapter] represent such a conversion [to bipolar disorder] is unknown* [emphasis added]." Notice in the italicized words how the FDA tries to cover its tracks while emphasizing this alleged side effect. Prior to 2004, the FDA and the pharmaceutical industry denied antidepressant-induced suicidality, insisting that suicidality resulted from the patients' underlying depression, in essence blaming the victims of this drug side effect. Now that the FDA has finally acknowledged antidepressants can make patients suicidal, the bipolar "spin" is the latest variation on the theme of blaming the victims.

With regard to stopping antidepressants when patients deteriorate or become suicidal on the drugs, the FDA notes: "If the decision is made to discontinue [antidepressant] treatment, [the] medication should be tapered, as rapidly as is feasible, but with recognition that abrupt discontinuation can be associated with certain symptoms," i.e., withdrawal reactions.[51] Guidelines for monitoring patients when lowering their antidepressant dose or tapering them off the drugs are included in the 5-Step Antidepressant Tapering Program discussed in the subsequent chapters of this book. Antidepressant-induced suicides and violence are almost completely preventable if patients are properly warned, monitored closely, and treated appropriately for any antidepressant-induced deterioration in their condition.

5

Worst Offenders

The Antidepressants that Cause the Most Frequent Withdrawal Reactions

Allison's Effexor Withdrawal After
Just One Missed Dose

A graduate student at Harvard's Kennedy School of Government, Allison felt "terrified" as she was wheeled out of her Wednesday afternoon seminar in the spring of 1999 on a stretcher and taken by ambulance to the hospital after she became dizzy, lightheaded, and faint in class. Just a year earlier, Allison's grandfather had died of a stroke. Am I having a stroke? Allison obsessed as the paramedics lifted her stretcher into the ambulance. Do strokes run in the family? The wail of the ambulance's siren, its flashing lights, and its high speed all aggravated Allison's dizziness, making her feel like she was going to pass out.

After five hours in the emergency room and multiple diagnostic tests, the doctors were baffled by Allison's case: They could find nothing wrong. The most likely diagnosis was a flu-type infection. But none of Allison's tests were abnormal, including her white blood count which one would expect to be abnormal if she had an infection. In the end, the doctors speculated that Allison was anxious because they could find no other explanation for her symptoms.

Allison protested that she had no history of anxiety and nothing in particular was stressing her at the time. She was in the second semester of a master's degree program that was going extremely well. She had a great job lined up for after graduation. She was in the middle of the semester; exams were on the distant horizon. She was not at all anxious about the particular seminar in which she had become ill.

Allison did have a history of depression and was on 100 milligrams of Effexor in the morning and again in the afternoon each day. "I felt a little resentful," says Allison of the emergency room doctors in retrospect. "I felt they were jumping to the conclusion that because I was on Effexor I was a psycho and must be anxious since they could find nothing else wrong." No one thought to ask Allison if she was taking her Effexor regularly.

Allison was sent home from the emergency room still feeling ill but reassured by the doctors that nothing serious like a stroke was happening to her. Allison's roommates came to the hospital to pick her up. At home, Allison could not eat any dinner; she had no appetite. She took her afternoon dose of Effexor on the late side, in the early evening, and went to bed. In the morning, she awoke feeling "miraculously" well. The dizziness, lightheadedness, and feeling faint were all gone. "That just made the whole thing more mysterious," says Allison. "What could I have had that made me feel so sick one day and was gone the next?"

Allison soon forgot the mysterious incident as she became caught up again in her busy life as a graduate student, until the same thing happened a month later. "I was actually sitting in the same early afternoon seminar when I started to feel ill again," Allison recounts. "This time I didn't say anything because I was afraid the professor would want to send me to the emergency room again. I just sat there preoccupied with wondering: What could this be? I knew I wasn't anxious. I never bought that idea. I systematically started taking an inventory of everything I'd eaten and done in the previous twenty-four hours, looking for clues to explain the mysterious symptoms. That's when it struck me: I hadn't taken my Effexor in the morning. Could that be it? I went straight home after class and took a dose in the mid-afternoon. Within three hours the symptoms were gone.

"I was angry that my family doctor hadn't warned me about Effexor withdrawal and that the doctors in the emergency room hadn't thought of it," says Allison. When Allison went to see her doctor, the doctor said she had never heard of Effexor withdrawal. Allison brought the doctor material on Effexor withdrawal that she found surfing the Web looking for information.[1] "I felt so odd educating my doctor about this," says Allison. "Isn't it supposed to be the other way around?" Many patients find themselves in this position, having to educate their doctors about antidepressant withdrawal and dependence.

A year later, in March 2000 the FDA required Effexor's manufacturer, Wyeth Pharmaceuticals, to add a new warning to their official information on the drug. The warning states that the antidepressant needs to be "tapered gradually" to reduce withdrawal reactions in "patients who have received Effexor for 6 weeks or more."[2] Effexor was introduced to the market in 1993, so it had been in use for seven years before the new warning was added. This was after numerous case reports of Effexor withdrawal, including reports published in medical journals of patients who, like Allison, had severe withdrawal reactions within hours of missing just one dose.[3] The warning goes on to say "the period required for tapering may depend on the dose, duration of therapy and the individual patient" but fails to give patients and doctors more detailed guidelines. In 2000, Wyeth became the first pharmaceutical company the FDA required to change its official information regarding withdrawal reactions with its drug. The same warning appears in Wyeth Pharmaceuticals' official information on Effexor XR, the slow-release form of the drug, since it does not provide protection from withdrawal.[4]

How do antidepressants cause withdrawal? Why would one antidepressant cause withdrawal reactions within hours of missing a dose, while other antidepressants do not cause withdrawal reactions for days or even weeks? Which antidepressants are the worst offenders—that is, cause withdrawal in the largest number of patients? Below are answers to these important questions, so you know what to expect with your particular antidepressant.

How Antidepressants Cause Withdrawal and Dependence

When patients start taking antidepressants, doctors typically advise them that the drugs can take up to a month to work, although side effects may occur sooner. The reason for bringing this to the attention of patients is so they will not become discouraged, especially if they develop side effects, and stop antidepressants after just a week or two. Many patients report that antidepressants only "kick in" after three or four weeks.

When patients go on antidepressants, their brain cells adapt, or change, in response to living with the drugs around the clock.[5] The adaptations take brain cells a month or more to complete. Some of the adaptations are believed responsible for the drugs' therapeutic effects. Since the adaptations can take a month to complete, the therapeutic effects may not develop for a month. Not all the adaptations brain cells make are therapeutic; others are believed responsible for the drugs' side effects.

In their adaptations, brain cells attempt to counteract the effects of antidepressants. One way of thinking about this is that brain cells do not like to be disturbed. Drugs are foreign substances in the brain and the cells react to try to protect their usual state. Doctors often tell patients that antidepressants increase serotonin signals in the brain. Serotonin is one of the chemical signals by which brain cells communicate with one another. To counteract the increase in serotonin signals, brain cells reduce their sensitivity to the signals in a process called "down regulation."[6] So, antidepressants are thought to put the signals up, brain cells compensate by putting the signals back down some, and a compromise is reached over the course of weeks or months.

Simple as that may sound, the adaptations are actually rather complex. They involve changes in the brain cells' receptors that pick up serotonin signals. Since the receptors are made of proteins, changes in protein synthesis occur within the cells. This involves changes in the instructions given by the cells' DNA, the master code regulating cellular function.[7] That is why the adaptations take weeks or months. Scientists do not yet fully understand how the adaptations brain cells make to antidepressants lead to their various therapeutic effects and side effects. This is an area of intense research. But we do know brain cells make significant adaptations to living with antidepressants 24/7 and maintain the adaptations for as long as patients are on the medications.

When patients stop taking antidepressants, their brain cells need to undo the adaptations they have made to living with the drugs, often for years. The cells need to *readapt* to living without the drugs. Whereas the cells down regulated when the drugs were introduced, now they need time to "up regulate" when the drugs are removed. Since the adaptations took weeks or months to put in place, they take weeks or months to dismantle. If the drugs are stopped abruptly, the brain cells do not have enough time to readapt; and the stress on the brain cells results in abnormal brain cell activity that produces the symptoms of antidepressant withdrawal. The same response happens, though to a lesser degree, if one simply lowers the dose: brain cells need sufficient time to readjust to the lower level of the drug.

Even when patients do not develop withdrawal symptoms following reductions in the dose of their antidepressants, their brain cells are still readjusting to the lower doses. The dosage reductions were just small enough so that they did not hit the threshold that would produce noticeable withdrawal symptoms in the particular patient. But the patients' brain cells are still readjusting, even though one does not see signs of the readjustment—that is, withdrawal symptoms.

Stopping an antidepressant or lowering the dose too abruptly is like driving a car at sixty miles an hour and suddenly throwing it into reverse. Instead, one slows the car down gradually, and only when it is stopped puts it in reverse. Similarly, with antidepressants one needs to gradually taper the drugs, allowing brain cells weeks to readapt to reasonable-sized dosage reductions.

Brain cells need sufficient time to readjust to a drop in the level of an antidepressant. This explains why restarting the drug or putting the dose back up suppresses withdrawal symptoms. If brain cells have not had enough time to readapt to a steep drop in the antidepressant, then restarting it or putting the dose back up reestablishes the drug level the brain cells are comfortable with. One then tapers off the drug more slowly to give brain cells the time they need to readjust.

Patients who have been on antidepressants less than a month typically do not experience withdrawal reactions if they stop the drug.[8] This, too, can be explained in terms of the adjustments and readjustments brain cells make to starting and stopping antidepressants. These patients' brain cells have typically not yet fully adapted to living with the drugs. So they have little to do in the way of readjusting if the drugs are stopped.

When patients take their last dose of an antidepressant, the drug does not simply disappear immediately from the body. Since patients have typically taken antidepressants for months or years, the drugs are distributed throughout the brain and the rest of the body. When patients stop an antidepressant, it "washes" out of the body by a variety of routes.[9] Some of it is excreted in the urine. Some of it is broken down, rendered inactive, by the liver. Similarly, when patients lower the dose of an antidepressant the excess drug level washes out. Antidepressants vary widely in how quickly or slowly they wash out of the body. We now understand that this is one of the crucial variables determining which antidepressants cause the most withdrawal.

How Quickly Antidepressants Wash Out of the Body

The technical, medical term for how quickly an antidepressant washes out of the body is its "half-life." I have tried to keep technical terms to a minimum, but this is one term you should know. An antidepressant's half-life is the length of time it takes for half the drug to wash out after one stops taking it. If the antidepressant's half-life is twenty-four hours, then twenty-four hours after the last dose—the next day—half the antidepressant is gone. By contrast, if an antidepressant's half-life is seven days, then it takes a week—instead of a day—for half of it to be eliminated. Obviously, this is a huge difference in terms of how gradually or precipitously the level of the drug drops and how much time brain cells have to readapt to the change. Another standard measure of how quickly antidepressants wash out is the time it takes for 90 percent of the drug to be eliminated from the body. Even after an antidepressant is gone, withdrawal symptoms can still persist because the brain cells are still distressed, trying to cope with the abrupt drop in the drug.

Table 5.1 lists the half-lives of today's antidepressants.[10] The table also lists how long it takes for 90 percent of each drug to be eliminated and the typical onset of withdrawal symptoms. The drugs are listed in order of how quickly they wash out of the body, from fastest to slowest. Effexor tops the list with an extremely short half-life of just five hours. Ninety percent of the drug is eliminated in a little more than a day. That is why patients can experience severe withdrawal symptoms within hours of missing just one dose.

Cymbalta, Luvox, Serzone, Paxil, Wellbutrin, Zoloft, Lexapro, Remeron, and Celexa also all have short half-lives of between twelve and thirty-five hours. Patients stopping these antidepressants typically develop withdrawal symptoms two to five days after stopping the drugs. When patients stop these other short-acting antidepressants, 90 percent is eliminated in three to seven days, depending on the particular drug.

As seen in Table 5.1, the "extended release" form of Effexor, Effexor XR, the "controlled release" form of Paxil, Paxil CR, and the "slow release" forms of Wellbutrin, Wellbutrin SR and Wellbutrin XL, all have the same or shorter half-lives as the original versions of the drugs. Some doctors mistakenly think these slow release versions of antidepressants protect against withdrawal reactions but this is not the case.[11] The slow

Table 5.1 THE HALF-LIVES, ELIMINATION TIMES,
AND TYPICAL ONSET OF WITHDRAWAL SYMPTOMS
AFTER STOPPING ANTIDEPRESSANTS

Antidepressant	Half-Life	90% Eliminated	Typical Onset of Withdrawal
Effexor	5 hours	1 day	Day 1–2
Effexor XR	5 hours	1 day	Day 1–2
Cymbalta	12 hours	2.5 days	Day 2–3
Luvox	15.6 hours	3.3 days	Day 2–3
Serzone	11–24 hours	3.6 days	Day 2–3
Paxil CR	15–20 hours	3.6 days	Day 2–3
Paxil	21 hours	4.4 days	Day 2–3
Wellbutrin	21 hours	4.4 days	Day 2–3
Wellbutrin SR Wellbutrin XL	21 hours	4.4 days	Day 2–3
Zoloft	26 hours	5.4 days	Day 3–4
Lexapro	27–32 hours	6.1 days	Day 3–5
Remeron	20–40 hours	6.3 days	Day 3–5
Celexa	35 hours	7.3 days	Day 3–6
Prozac	4–6 days	25 days	2–3 weeks

release mechanism affects how the antidepressant is released from the pill into the stomach and blood stream. But slow release determines how quickly or slowly an antidepressant *enters* the body; rather than how quickly or slowly the drug *washes out* when it is stopped or the dose is lowered.

In Table 5.1, Prozac is set off from the other antidepressants because it has a much longer half-life, four to six days. It takes more than three weeks for 90 percent of Prozac to be eliminated from the body. Because Prozac has this slow, built-in taper, withdrawal reactions are less common with Prozac than other antidepressants.

The frequency with which antidepressants cause withdrawal reactions correlates with how short their half-lives are. Table 5.2 shows the results of a pair of studies done at the Massachusetts General Hospital and Harvard Medical School investigating the frequency of withdrawal reactions with Effexor, Paxil, Zoloft, and Prozac.[12] Effexor causes withdrawal reactions in an extremely high percentage of patients, 78 percent. Paxil and Zoloft are close behind with 66 and 60 percent of patients, respectively. Prozac causes withdrawal reactions in 14 percent of patients. Notice in Table 5.2 that the rank order of frequency of withdrawal reactions correlates with the half-lives of these antidepressants. That is, the shorter-acting antidepressants cause more withdrawal symptoms. This is because the frequency with which antidepressants cause withdrawal reactions correlates with how quickly they wash out of the body.

Effexor is the worst offender in terms of the lightning speed with which it can cause withdrawal reactions. Patients who miss their morning dose of Effexor can find themselves in the throes of withdrawal reactions by late morning.[13] Patients who miss their evening dose can be awoken in the middle of the night by withdrawal symptoms.[14] Some patients report feeling "held hostage" by their Effexor dose; if they fail to take it like clockwork they can be in withdrawal within an hour or two of a missed dose.

Prozac causes withdrawal symptoms in 14 percent of patients, in marked contrast to the much higher rates for the shorter-acting antidepressants. But, 14 percent of patients is still quite a lot. A side effect that occurs in more than 1 percent of patients is officially considered a frequent side effect.[15] One of the big surprises in the large-scale, systematic studies of antidepressant withdrawal reactions done in the mid- to late-1990s is that antidepressant withdrawal reactions are *not* rare with

Table 5.2 FREQUENCY OF ANTIDEPRESSANT WITHDRAWAL REACTIONS

ANTIDEPRESSANT	HALF-LIFE	FREQUENCY OF WITHDRAWAL REACTIONS
Effexor	5 hours	78%
Paxil	21 hours	66%
Zoloft	26 hours	60%
Prozac	4–6 days	14%

Prozac when one carefully evaluates patients for withdrawal symptoms. When Prozac causes withdrawal symptoms, the onset tends to be later—up to twenty-five days after stopping the drug in published reports—and the symptoms tend to last longer—up to fifty-six days.[16] Therefore, even patients on Prozac should taper off of it carefully if they are taking doses of more than 20 milligrams a day.

Although Prozac is still generally considered to be less problematic than the other antidepressants when it comes to withdrawal reactions, some psychiatrists question this.[17] The percentages of patients experiencing Prozac, Zoloft, and Paxil withdrawal symptoms are based on a large-scale study of over two hundred patients.[18] In the study, patients stopped their antidepressants and were assessed for withdrawal symptoms for up to eight days. While eight days may be long enough to detect most Paxil or Zoloft withdrawal reactions, Prozac withdrawal symptoms can take weeks to appear. Since the researchers only assessed patients for eight days, many cases of Prozac withdrawal reactions may have been missed, making it likely that the 14 percent figure for Prozac is an underestimate.[19]

Moreover, diagnosing Prozac withdrawal reactions is complicated by the increased risk of confusing it with depressive relapse, a return of patients' original psychiatric conditions.[20] Since the other antidepressants typically cause withdrawal symptoms within days of stopping the drug or lowering the dose, this makes it easier to separate withdrawal reactions from depressive relapse, which occurs later as discussed in the previous chapter. But, the later onset and longer duration of Prozac withdrawal reactions make them more difficult to distinguish from depressive relapse. This increases the risk of the antidepressant catch-22 for patients on Prozac: the risk of withdrawal reactions being misdiagnosed as depressive relapse and patients needlessly being put back on the drug. This is an aspect of antidepressant withdrawal that still needs more research.

How Antidepressants Affect Brain Chemicals

Most patients on SSRI-type antidepressants have been told these drugs are "selective" for the brain chemical serotonin. Indeed, many patients are told that they correct a "biochemical imbalance," enhancing serotonin signals in the brain to correct a serotonin deficiency allegedly responsible for depression. However, antidepressants do not exclusively affect serotonin.[21] Moreover, there is no proof of a biochemical imbalance, a serotonin deficiency, in depression.[22] Experts now scoff at the idea that the drugs do anything so simple. Indeed, in Ireland and other countries, the regulatory agencies equivalent to our FDA have forced pharmaceutical companies to stop claiming antidepressants correct serotonin deficiencies in their advertising and marketing promotions of the drugs.[23]

Antidepressants affect other brain chemicals directly and indirectly to varying degrees.[24] Paxil in particular blocks a group of receptors in the nervous system known as "cholinergic" receptors, producing what are called "anticholinergic" side effects.[25] When Paxil is stopped, reversal of these effects produces a condition known as "cholinergic rebound" which may exacerbate Paxil withdrawal.[26] A number of experts believe this is still another reason why Paxil is one of the worst offenders: because of the particular constellation of brain chemicals that it affects.

How Widely an Antidepressant Is Prescribed

Another major factor determining which antidepressants are the worst offenders is how widely prescribed each of the drugs is. Over the last decade, the three best-selling antidepressants have been Prozac, Paxil, and Zoloft. The original drug, Prozac, has now gone off patent, meaning Eli Lilly no longer has the exclusive rights to it. Instead, Prozac has become generic, so any drug company can now manufacture it. Since Eli Lilly no longer has any reason to promote Prozac, its sales have plummeted.

In 2000—just before Prozac went off patent—Prozac, Paxil, and Zoloft were all in the top ten best selling of all drugs of any kind for the year. Prozac ranked number six with sales of $2.9 billion.[27] Paxil ranked seventh with sales of $2.4 billion and Zoloft ranked eighth with sales of $2.2 billion. Table 5.3 summarizes their sales in billions of dollars. By 2002 the situation was a little different because Prozac had gone off patent and dropped off the list of the top ten best-selling drugs while Paxil and Zoloft remained multibillion-dollar best sellers.

Of the three best selling antidepressants, Paxil and Zoloft are the two with short half-lives, washing out of the body precipitously and causing a high percentage of patients to have withdrawal reactions. By comparison with these drugs, the other antidepressants with short half-lives have been prescribed to fewer patients. In terms of sheer numbers—people affected by antidepressant withdrawal reactions—Paxil and Zoloft are the

Table 5.3 BEST-SELLING ANTIDEPRESSANTS IN 2000

ANTIDEPRESSANT	RANK AMONG BEST-SELLING DRUGS	DOLLAR SALES
Prozac	6	$2.9 billion
Paxil	7	$2.4 billion
Zoloft	8	$2.2 billion

BEST-SELLING ANTIDEPRESSANTS IN 2002

ANTIDEPRESSANT	RANK AMONG BEST-SELLING DRUGS	DOLLAR SALES
Paxil	8	$3.3 billion
Zoloft	10	$2.9 billion
Prozac	Generic; no longer a best seller	

worst offenders. Of course, individual patients on the other short-acting antidepressants (all the antidepressants except Prozac) have a high chance of developing withdrawal symptoms if they stop the drugs or make too large a reduction in the doses. But the total number of patients affected is lower because these drugs are prescribed to fewer patients.

While I was writing this book, the patent for Paxil expired. The patent for Zoloft is due to expire. If another antidepressant becomes one of the top ten best-selling drugs, then it, too, could cause withdrawal reactions in significant numbers of patients. In fact, Forest Laboratories pharmaceutical company has been aggressively promoting Celexa and Eli Lilly has been aggressively promoting Cymbalta as the new kids on the block.[28] If Celexa or Cymbalta become best-selling drugs, they could cause withdrawal reactions in large numbers of patients. However, it may be that none of the other antidepressants in this group will make it to the ranks of the best sellers because they are no longer viewed as miracle cures. Rather, doctors and patients are increasingly familiar with their limitations and side effects.

How Antidepressants Are Promoted

One last variable seems to have made Paxil the worst offender in the minds of many patients; that is the way in which Paxil has been aggressively marketed by GlaxoSmithKline in direct-to-consumer advertisements and brochures as "non-habit forming," "not associated with dependence or addiction," and causing "mild, usually temporary, side effects."[29] According to many of my patients, this intangible factor cannot be underestimated.

Reporters doing articles or shows on antidepressants often ask me: Why do I hear so much about Paxil withdrawal? Doesn't Zoloft withdrawal affect almost as many people? What about Effexor, which can cause withdrawal after just one missed dose? What about all the other antidepressants that cause high rates of withdrawal? Why are patients so upset over Paxil withdrawal? I think the answer lies in the misleading television advertisements and brochures aimed at patients. One of the reasons class action lawsuits have been filed over Paxil withdrawal and not yet other antidepressants is the tremendous anger patients feel going through months of Paxil withdrawal all the while watching the television advertisements claiming the drug is non-habit forming.

Preparing patients and their families for side effects has an impact on how they react to them. If patients are warned of side effects, they know what to expect. When patients are not warned, the surprise element compounds their pain and suffering. They feel blindsided, which makes them more upset. But if patients feel *misled,* they do not just feel surprised: they feel betrayed. This can leave them enraged. Family members feel much the same way if they are affected by patients' withdrawal symptoms, for example, having to cope with their irritability. When they feel betrayed, the anger patients and families feel over antidepressant withdrawal reactions can last for years after the withdrawal has cleared. The resulting anger can damage the public trust of doctors, the medical profession, and the health care system in general.

The Worst Offenders

In summary, Paxil and Zoloft are the worst offenders in terms of the sheer numbers of people affected by withdrawal reactions, because they are short acting and have been widely prescribed. Effexor is the worst offender in terms of the lightning speed with which it can cause withdrawal reactions, within hours of just one missed dose. The other short-acting antidepressants—Celexa, Lexapro, Luvox, Wellbutrin, Cymbalta, Remeron, and Serzone—can still cause withdrawal in a high percentage of patients. And the withdrawal reactions can be severe, as in Karen's life-threatening Celexa withdrawal in the previous chapter. Prozac causes the fewest withdrawal reactions, because its long half-life provides a slow, built-in taper.

6

The 5-Step Antidepressant Tapering Program
How to Avoid Uncomfortable or Dangerous Withdrawal Reactions

The best way to minimize antidepressant withdrawal reactions is to carefully taper, or wean, off the drugs with close medical supervision. Although tapering can reduce the severity of withdrawal symptoms, it does not necessarily eliminate them altogether. Many patients will still have withdrawal symptoms even with slow tapers. But the symptoms are less severe than if the patients suddenly stopped their antidepressants.

The 5-Step Antidepressant Tapering Program is summarized in Table 6.1 and briefly described below to give you an overview of the program before looking more closely at each step in subsequent chapters.

Step 1: Evaluating Whether You Are Ready to Try Tapering Off Your Antidepressant

The first step in an antidepressant tapering program is deciding whether you are, in fact, ready to try tapering off the drug. This is a decision made collaboratively by the doctor and patient after careful consideration. As part of such an evaluation one considers: Has the patient's original depression or other psychiatric condition improved enough and for long enough to consider going off the medication? Has the patient grown psychologically in ways that make him less vulnerable to depression either

Table 6.1 THE 5-STEP ANTIDEPRESSANT TAPERING PROGRAM

Step 1: Evaluating whether you are ready to try tapering off your
    antidepressant

Step 2: Making the initial dosage reduction

Step 3: Monitoring withdrawal symptoms after a dosage reduction

Step 4: Making additional dosage reductions

Step 5: The end-of-taper evaluation

---

through psychotherapy, couples therapy, cognitive-behavioral treatment, a twelve-step program, or some other treatment modality that has
addressed the underlying problem? Have the patient's life circumstances
changed such that the set of circumstances that originally made her depressed are no longer present? Does the patient have side effects prompting a desire to go off the drug? Does the patient have such severe side
effects that she has no choice but to go off the drug? Even if the patient
has no side effects, does she want to go off the drug rather than stay on it
indefinitely because of concerns about the long-term, largely unknown
side effects and risks?

Sometimes after completing such an evaluation, the patient decides
that he is not yet ready to go off the antidepressant. If the patient still
needs an antidepressant but has significant side effects, sometimes an alternative strategy is used, such as lowering the dose to see if the side effect
improves or switching to another antidepressant in a different class. If the
patient's circumstances are favorable for going off the antidepressant,
then one proceeds to the next step in the 5-Step Antidepressant Tapering
Program.

Step 2: Making the Initial Dosage Reduction

Table 6.2 presents the series of recommended dosage reductions in the
5-Step Antidepressant Tapering Program for each of today's popular
antidepressants. The programs in Table 6.2 are based on extensive experience tapering patients off antidepressants. The suggested dosage reductions are carefully chosen to be comfortable in size for the majority of

patients; that is, to produce mild withdrawal reactions or no withdrawal reactions at all, although this varies with individuals.

Working with your doctor to determine the recommended tapering program for you, find the dose of your antidepressant in the table and review the series of suggested dosage reductions to taper off the drug. These may need to be adjusted following the guidelines of the 5-Step Antidepressant Tapering Program, particularly if you have moderate to severe withdrawal reactions. As seen in Table 6.2, if you are on 20 milligrams a day of Paxil, the suggested initial dosage reduction is from 20 to 10 milligrams a day. If you are on 150 milligrams a day of Zoloft, the recommended initial dosage reduction is from 150 to 100 milligrams a day. If you are on 150 milligrams a day of Effexor, the suggested initial dosage reduction is from 150 to 75 milligrams a day. Patients who should proceed more slowly than the recommended tapering programs, are discussed in Chapter 8: Making the Initial Dosage Reduction.

Notice in Table 6.2 that antidepressants are prescribed in different increments. Whereas a Paxil taper may go from 60 to 40 to 20 to 10 to 0, an Effexor taper may go from 225 to 150 to 75 to 37.5 to 0.

Subsequent chapters will examine six patients' tapering programs in detail to illustrate how the 5-Step Antidepressant Tapering Program works. The six patients—Claudia, Richard, Sarah, Gary, Daria, and Brent—all taper off 20 milligrams a day of Paxil. They all make the same initial dosage reduction from 20 down to 10 milligrams a day. I chose six patients on Paxil because when discussing antidepressant withdrawal, Paxil is often used as the reference drug since it is most frequently associated with withdrawal symptoms. I chose six patients on the same dose because they illustrate the wide range of withdrawal reactions possible in different patients tapering off the same dose of an antidepressant.

Step 3: Monitoring Withdrawal Symptoms After a Dosage Reduction

Following a dosage reduction, one to three appointments are set up to evaluate and monitor the patient's withdrawal symptoms. The appointments are scheduled to coincide with when withdrawal symptoms are most likely to appear. Using a daily checklist (see Appendix 1), doctors and patients keep track of when withdrawal symptoms appear and their time course. By closely monitoring a patient, the pattern of the patient's

Table 6.2 RECOMMENDED TAPERING PROGRAMS FOR TODAY'S POPULAR ANTIDEPRESSANTS

Working with your doctor, find the dose of your antidepressant in the table below and review the series of suggested dosage reductions to taper off the drug. These dosage reductions may need to be adjusted following the guidelines of the 5-Step Antidepressant Tapering Program, particularly if you have moderate to severe withdrawal reactions. All doses are in milligrams/day. Note: See Chapter 12 for guidelines on adjusting the dosage reductions for children and adolescents.

Paxil	Paxil CR	Zoloft	Celexa	Lexapro	Luvox	Prozac	Effexor / Effexor XR	Serzone	Cymbalta	Remeron	Wellbutrin / Wellbutrin XL	Wellbutrin SR	Zyban
		200				80							
60	50	150	40	20	300	60	225	600	60	45	450	400	300
40	25	100	20	10	200	40	150	400	40	30	300	300	150
20	12.5	50	10	5	100	20	75	200	20	15	150	150	75
10	0	25	0	0	50	0	37.5	100	10	7.5	75	75	0
0		0			0		0	0	0	0	0	0	

SSRIs (Paxil, Paxil CR, Zoloft, Celexa, Lexapro, Luvox, Prozac) | *SNRIs* (Effexor / Effexor XR, Serzone, Cymbalta, Remeron) | *Other* (Wellbutrin / Wellbutrin XL, Wellbutrin SR, Zyban) withdrawal reaction is established. That pattern traces the onset, peak, resolution, and severity of withdrawal symptoms. If the symptoms become intolerable, the dose of the antidepressant is put back up and the tapering schedule is extended. Of the six patients followed in detail in subsequent chapters, after their initial dosage reductions, two have little or no withdrawal reactions, two have moderate withdrawal reactions, and two have severe withdrawal reactions.

Step 4: Making Additional Dosage Reductions

When the initial dosage reduction in your antidepressant tapering program is made, you usually have no idea how you are going to react, that is, how mild or severe a withdrawal reaction you are going to have. But, when making additional dosage reductions, the severity of your withdrawal reaction to the previous reduction determines the size of the next reduction. Following the recommended dosage reductions in the 5-Step Antidepressant Tapering Program, most patients have mild withdrawal reactions or no withdrawal reactions at all. Under these circumstances, you can continue to follow the tapering program—the recommended dosage reductions—in Table 6.2. On the other hand, if you have a moderate or severe withdrawal reaction, then you will need to try smaller dosage reductions—following the guidelines in Chapter 10 for customizing dosage reductions—until you find a comfortable size dosage reduction that you can repeat; that is, one that causes mild withdrawal reactions or no withdrawal reaction at all.

Dosage reductions are made every three to five weeks, about once a month. This allows time for whatever withdrawal symptoms you experience to peak and subside, and it leaves time for you to fully recover from an episode of withdrawal. Even if you do not experience any withdrawal symptoms, you should wait this long to allow your brain cells time to fully adjust to the lower dose before reducing it further. Making repeated, more frequent dosage reductions produces a cumulative effect of rapidly lowering the level of the drug in the brain that can "catch up" with you and increase the risk of more severe withdrawal reactions. As you progress through an antidepressant tapering program, you establish a routine of alternating between making dosage reductions and monitoring episodes of withdrawal symptoms.

This routine continues until the final reduction when you stop the drug. While the pattern of a patient's withdrawal symptoms—their onset, peak, resolution, and severity—is likely to repeat itself with each dosage reduction of comparable size, this may not hold true as one gets to lower and lower doses near the end of a taper. Sometimes, in the final stages of a tapering program, one has to make smaller reductions, to minimize worsening symptoms.

Table 6.3 shows the dosage reductions of the six patients whose tapering programs we will be examining in detail. Claudia and Richard had few or no withdrawal reactions and were able to follow the recommended tapering program for patients on 20 milligrams a day of Paxil— that is, 20 to 10 to 0 milligrams a day. Sarah and Gary had moderate withdrawal reactions and had to slow their tapers down, making 5 and 2.5-milligram reductions. Daria had a severe withdrawal reaction and had to taper painstakingly slowly, making dosage reductions of 2.5 milligrams at a time. Brent had the hardest time of all. His reaction was so severe when he reduced his daily dose from 20 to 10 milligrams that he was forced to put the dose back up. He had another severe withdrawal reaction when he tried reducing his daily dose from 20 to 15 milligrams. Thereafter, he reduced his daily dose painstakingly slowly by 2.5 milligrams at a time roughly every three weeks. As seen in Table 6.3, these six patients illustrate the wide range of withdrawal reactions seen in patients tapering off the same dose of an antidepressant.

Claudia, Richard, Sarah, Gary, Daria, and Brent were chosen to illustrate the wide range of possible withdrawal reactions to tapering off the same dose of an antidepressant. Whereas Claudia and Richard completed their tapering program in just six weeks, Brent's took six and a half months. The 5-Step Antidepressant Tapering Program is a flexible approach that recommends a tapering program for each antidepressant and, at the same time, provides guidelines for adjusting the program, for making smaller dosage reductions, if necessary. Following the program's guidelines, in my experience most patients have no withdrawal reaction at all or mild withdrawal reactions that they tolerate comfortably, like Claudia and Richard. Few patients have withdrawal reactions so severe they are forced to go back up on the dose as Brent did.

Step 5: The End-of-Taper Evaluation

The final dosage reduction—when the patient stops the antidepressant altogether—may produce withdrawal symptoms that are more severe since the drug is now completely washing out of the patient's system.

Table 6.3 THE TAPERING PROGRAMS OF SIX PATIENTS
GOING OFF 20 MILLIGRAMS A DAY OF PAXIL

Claudia and Richard were able to follow the recommended tapering program (Table 6.2) for patients on 20 milligrams a day of Paxil, reducing their daily dose from 20 to 10 to 0 milligrams, making dosage reductions about once a month. The other patients had to slow their tapers down, because of moderate or severe withdrawal reactions, making smaller reductions roughly once a month.

RECOMMENDED	Claudia	Richard	Sarah	Gary	Daria	Brent
20	20	20	20	20	20	20
10	10	10	10	10	10	10
0	0	0	5	5	7.5	20
			0	2.5	5	15
				0	2.5	12.5
					0	10
						7.5
						5
						2.5
						0

Patients should continue to be monitored just as they had been after earlier dosage reductions. The taper should not be considered over until the patient has fully recovered from whatever withdrawal symptoms occur after stopping the drug. If the patient has incapacitating withdrawal symptoms after stopping the drug altogether, then the last dose is reinstated and one or two smaller dosage reductions are used to finish the taper.

Advanced Planning

As part of preparing patients to enter an antidepressant tapering program, patients should be asked to count out their remaining pills prior to meeting to plan the initial dosage reduction. One patient may have ten of the 20-milligram Paxil pills left and two refills waiting to be filled while another patient may only have a few pills. As the dose is lowered, patients may have to cut pills in half or even quarters to achieve lower doses so the doctor needs to know what size pills and how many they have.

During the tapering program, patients and doctors need to meet regularly to plan dosage reductions and monitor withdrawal symptoms. Typically, about three appointments are required each month. Family doctors who do not feel they have the time in their schedules or do not feel they have the expertise can refer patients to specialists.

Frequently Asked Questions and Answers

When I start patients on antidepressant tapering programs or when I make presentations on tapering the drugs to groups of clinicians, a number of common questions arise.

Question: Can antidepressants be taken every other day as part of tapering off them?

Answer: None of the short-acting antidepressants should be taken every other day as a way of tapering them. Because of their short half-lives, the every other day schedule can result in roller coaster levels of the drugs and roller coaster episodes of withdrawal symptoms.[1] This is true for Paxil, Zoloft, Celexa, Lexapro, Luvox, Effexor, Cymbalta, Serzone, Remeron, and Wellbutrin. Since Prozac is long-acting, it is the one antidepressant that can be taken every other day as part of tapering the drug. Because of Prozac's long half-life, patients on every other day schedules typically do not notice any difference between the days when they take a dose and the days when they do not. Because Prozac lingers so long in the body, the fluctuations in the level of the drug are typically not great enough to produce withdrawal symptoms. For most patients, taking 20 milligrams of Prozac every other day is equivalent to taking 10 milligrams a day. Occasionally, patients taking Prozac every other day will notice the difference and then one can return to daily dosing. But with all the other antidepressants, every other day dosing should be avoided.

Question: When pacing an antidepressant taper, is it better to err on the side of going a little faster or a little slower?

Answer: In general, one does not want to taper antidepressants either too slowly or too quickly. Tapering too slowly needlessly prolongs the process for patients. On the other hand, tapering too quickly leads to distressing, potentially incapacitating or even dangerous withdrawal symptoms. One tries to strike a balance. When in doubt, erring on the side of taking a little more time enhances the likelihood that the process will go smoothly. This ensures patients remain comfortable and provides a psychological cushion as well, giving patients a little more time to adjust to the idea of doing without drugs they have relied on. After a patient has been on an antidepressant for years, taking an extra month or two to ensure his comfort level is well worth the time. One hears stories of patients getting "stuck" part of the way through antidepressant tapers—being unable to go below a threshold dose of their drug. One also hears stories of patients having to go back on antidepressants shortly after stopping them. Often patients get "stuck" on antidepressants or have to go right back on them because they were not weaned slowly enough off the drugs to allow adequate time for their brain cells to readjust and to allow them adequate time to psychologically adjust to living without the drugs.

Question: Can antidepressant withdrawal symptoms do any injury to the brain or to other organ systems?

Answer: We assume that withdrawal symptoms do not cause injury to brain cells or to other organ systems. But, since it has not been adequately researched, we do not really know the answer to this question. The question is often asked by patients with severe symptoms like electric "zap" sensations in their brains or disabling withdrawal symptoms. Because we lack a definitive answer, patients should be discouraged from repeatedly "toughing out" severe withdrawal symptoms. Instead, the tapering schedule should be paced so that patients experience mild, tolerable withdrawal symptoms. This provides something of an "insurance policy" since we do not really know the answer to this important question.

Question: Instead of tapering a short-acting antidepressant, might one switch to another, longer-acting antidepressant to provide some built-in taper?

Answer: When antidepressant withdrawal reactions emerged as a serious problem with these drugs, some experts recommended switching from one antidepressant to another for this reason. But this has not become a widely used strategy because of a number of problems. While switching antidepressants worked in some published cases, it did not work in others, making it a risky, unreliable approach to coping with antidepressant withdrawal.[2] Moreover, since patients respond differently to different antidepressants, introducing a change in drug may introduce a whole new set of side effects. Finally, Prozac has the longest half-life, but even Prozac should be tapered from doses higher than 20 milligrams a day. As discussed in the previous chapter, the delayed onset and longer duration of withdrawal symptoms with Prozac can make it more difficult to distinguish withdrawal reactions from relapses, increasing the risk of the antidepressant catch-22. For all these reasons, switching antidepressants is not a good strategy.

Question: If one gets "stuck" on a low dose of an antidepressant—that is, one is unable to go down to lower doses because of severe withdrawal reactions—can adding a low dose of Prozac help?

Answer: I have not had to resort to this strategy because the tapering schedules I have used in the 5-Step Antidepressant Tapering Program have succeeded without doing so. However, a number of my colleagues have told me that adding a low dose of Prozac (for example, 10 milligrams a day) has been helpful for patients who became "stuck" on a low dose of one of the other selective serotonin reuptake inhibitors (SSRIs) or serotonin and noradrenalin reuptake inhibitors (SNRIs) (see Table 6.2 on page 93). Note that this is *adding* a low dose of Prozac, not *substituting*, or switching to, Prozac, as discussed above. Once the Prozac is established, one finishes tapering the original antidepressant. Then one stops the Prozac with its slow, built-in taper. I have the same reservations about adding Prozac that I have about switching to it, because this introduces another potent prescription drug into the mix, and one has no way of knowing how a patient will react to it. However, it may be worth resorting to in difficult, intractable cases. One only stops the Prozac after the patient has completely tapered off the original antidepressant.

Question: What if a person is on two or more antidepressants at the same time, a so-called antidepressant "cocktail"?

Answer: Antidepressant "cocktails" have become popular with psychopharmacologists—psychiatrists who just prescribe medications and do not typically do psychotherapy—in the past decade. When patients are on two or more antidepressants, they have two choices: taper completely off one of the antidepressants before beginning to taper off the other or taper the two simultaneously, alternating dosage reductions between the two. If the patient and doctor feel relatively confident that the patient no longer needs any antidepressant, then they may elect to taper both at the same time, alternating dosage reductions between the two. If one does this, one should alternate dosage reductions and not reduce the two simultaneously to avoid confusion about which drug is causing which withdrawal symptoms. Some patients feel that one antidepressant is no longer helping or is causing intolerable side effects, while the other antidepressant may still be helping. These patients may elect to taper one antidepressant and see how they do off of it before considering tapering the other one.

Question: Are there treatments for specific antidepressant withdrawal symptoms?

Answer: Some experts recommend additional drugs to treat specific antidepressant withdrawal symptoms, such as prescription sleeping pills for insomnia or antiemetics for vomiting.[3] In general, I do not like to use additional drugs to treat drug side effects, in this case withdrawal side effects. Some patients use over-the-counter remedies like Tylenol for withdrawal-induced headaches. Some patients use herbal sedatives or Benadryl for withdrawal-induced insomnia. Others use over-the-counter motion sickness medications—like Dramamine or Bonnine—for withdrawal-induced dizziness and imbalance. Still other patients use acupuncture or herbal preparations like ginger root for severe nausea.[4] Most of my patients prefer to find dosage reductions that are comfortable without having to resort even to over-the-counter remedies. Most patients have been able to accomplish this.

The problem with using potent prescription drugs to treat antidepressant withdrawal symptoms is that they come with their own set of side effects. Prescription sleeping pills, for example, cause rebound insomnia when they are stopped. Moreover, patients can become dependent on them. Antidepressant withdrawal symptoms represent stress on the nervous system, brain cells trying to readjust to lower levels of the drug. The severity of the symptoms can be a valuable gauge of the degree of stress on the nervous system. Blunting antidepressant withdrawal symptoms with prescription drugs distorts and obscures this gauge. Severe withdrawal symptoms are an important signal to slow the taper down in order to ease the stress. I prefer to slow the taper rather than mask the stress with other drugs.

Using additional drugs to treat antidepressant withdrawal symptoms was not a routine part of tapering earlier classes of antidepressants. Some doctors tell me that they resorted to using additional drugs to blunt withdrawal symptoms with today's popular antidepressants because they did not know what else to do. They did not fully understand that withdrawal symptoms represent brain cells needing more time to adjust to lower levels of the drug. And they lacked adequate training in how to slow the taper down enough to make patients comfortable and give their brain cells sufficient time to readjust. One key to success is taking the necessary time to taper. When one does not take sufficient time, patients are much more likely to get "stuck" on a low dose or feel like they need to return to a higher dose.

7

Step 1: Evaluating Whether You Are Ready to Try Tapering Off Your Antidepressant

Today's popular antidepressants are called "antidepressants" only because they were first approved for the treatment of depression. Since then their use has expanded to numerous other conditions. Antidepressants are now regularly prescribed for anxiety, shyness, worrying, social anxiety, obsessions, compulsions, posttraumatic stress, eating disorders, impulsivity, gambling, back pain, headaches, drug and alcohol abuse, premenstrual syndrome, premature ejaculation, attention deficit disorder, sexual addictions, irritability, hair pulling, nail biting, upset stomach, and chronic fatigue syndrome. Indeed, some doctors even suggest them for patients with no psychiatric conditions, to feel "better than well," a practice I do not support.[1] With so many antidepressants being used for such a large number of conditions, this chapter cannot cover every possible set of circumstances in which a patient might consider going off an antidepressant. Instead, I will discuss the key criteria one examines, which are summarized in Table 7.1, and use case examples to illustrate the points.

Preferably, the person meets both criteria 1 and 2:

1. *The patient's original condition has improved substantially.* Ideally, the patient is free of symptoms of the condition; that is, in complete remission. Of course, one typically does not go off an antidepressant the

Table 7.1 KEY CRITERIA FOR ESTABLISHING THAT A
PATIENT IS READY TO TRY GOING OFF AN ANTIDEPRESSANT

Preferably, the patient meets both criteria 1 and 2.

1. The patient's original condition has improved substantially.
2. The patient is in a relatively stable, calm period in life.

In addition, preferably the patient meets one or both of criteria 3 and 4.

3. The patient has grown, or changed, psychologically in ways that make her less vulnerable to the condition the drug was used to treat.
4. The patient's life circumstances have changed so significantly that the circumstances originally making him depressed, anxious, or otherwise symptomatic are no longer present.

In addition, meeting criteria 5 and 6 adds further weight to the decision.

5. The patient has significant side effects that contribute to the desire to go off the medication or that necessitate going off.
6. The patient wants to go off the antidepressant rather than stay on it indefinitely because of concerns about long-term, largely unknown, side effects and risks, especially if she no longer needs the drug.

---

minute one is feeling better. The general guideline is that when patients feel an antidepressant has helped, they should wait until they have been on the drug at least six months before trying to go off. Some patients feel in retrospect that they were prescribed antidepressants needlessly for the stresses and strains of everyday life rather than legitimate psychiatric conditions. When this is the case, the patient may have only had quite mild symptoms to begin with.

2. *The patient is in a relatively stable, calm period in life.* When one embarks on an antidepressant tapering program, one wants to pick an optimal time to do so. One tries to avoid stressful periods of transition or crisis that may undermine the effort to wean off.

In addition to meeting criteria 1 and 2, preferably the patient also meets one or both of criteria 3 and 4:

3. *The patient has grown, or changed, psychologically in ways that make her less vulnerable to the condition the drug was used to treat.* The psychological growth may have been achieved through psychotherapy, couples therapy, cognitive-behavioral treatment, twelve-step programs, disciplined exercise, spiritual renewal, or another treatment or self-help modality aimed at addressing the underlying problem. I include twelve-step programs, disciplined exercise, and spiritual renewal because psychiatrists like myself and other psychotherapists do not have an exclusive franchise on helping people help themselves. Twelve-step programs are among the most effective forms of treatment for substance abuse and other addictions. Studies have shown that for some people exercise can be as effective for depression as antidepressant drugs.[2] And some people find the path out of depression or other conditions through spiritual practices.

Some patients have been told their underlying problem is a serotonin deficiency that is corrected by an antidepressant. But this has never been proven, and in other countries the equivalents of our FDA have banned pharmaceutical companies from making this misleading claim.[3] Patients are also often told their psychiatric conditions are genetic, even though this, too, has not been proven.[4] Reports that genes have been found for psychiatric conditions have not stood the test of time. Even high profile, widely publicized reports have later been quietly retracted.[5] Patients are often told their psychiatric condition is a "disease." In fact, no psychiatric condition is a disease.[6] Strict criteria exist in medicine for calling conditions diseases (i.e. the cause of the condition or an understanding of its physiology must be established), and no psychiatric condition meets these criteria. This is why the official name for depression in the American Psychiatric Association's *Diagnostic and Statistical Manual of Mental Disorders (DSM)* is "major depressive *disorder*" not "major depressive disease."[7] Depression is a psychological condition, not a medical disease. Finally, some patients are told depression is a "life-long disease" so they should take their drugs indefinitely. But, experts point out that before the heavy marketing of antidepressant drugs in the 1990s, for centuries all but the most severe depressions were viewed as self-limiting conditions that typically resolved spontaneously without drug treatment in less than six months.[8] As described in Chapter 4, experts refer to the pharmaceutical industry's promoting the idea of psychiatric conditions as diseases, even lifelong diseases, as "marketing diseases to market drugs." Few patients are told this "disease model" is hypothetical and driven largely by the marketing of drugs. Instead, patients are often given the impression that it is a fully established, scientific fact. Patients need help counterbalancing these misleading ideas, which have become pervasive in our culture in the last decade, when evaluating whether they are ready to try going off their antidepressants.

4. *The patient's life circumstances have changed so significantly that the circumstances originally making him depressed, anxious, or otherwise symptomatic are no longer present.* Examples of dramatic improvement in a patient's circumstances that can contribute to his being less vulnerable to becoming depressed or anxious again if he goes off his medication are: settling into a new job after a difficult period of being unemployed, graduating from a stressful degree program, getting out of an abusive relationship, mourning a loss, or achieving success that counters an earlier blow to self-esteem.

Finally, meeting criteria 5 and/or 6 adds further weight to the decision to try going off an antidepressant:

5. *The patient has significant side effects that contribute to the desire to go off the medication or that necessitate going off.* Sexual dysfunction and weight gain are two of the most common reasons why patients want to go off today's antidepressants. Patients with significant side effects who have met several or all of the above criteria will probably want to try going off their antidepressant to obtain relief from the side effects. Patients with significant side effects who have not met enough of the above criteria may elect to stay with the antidepressant or switch to one in a different class less likely to cause the particular side effect. But when the new antidepressant is in a different class, the old antidepressant still needs to be tapered since the new one will not protect against withdrawal from the old one. Severe side effects—like Karen's antidepressant toxicity in Chapter 4—force some patients to go off the drugs.

6. *The patient wants to go off the antidepressant rather than stay on it indefinitely because of concerns about long-term, largely unknown side effects and risks.* While the risks may not be known with certainty, this is a legitimate concern, especially if the patient no longer needs the drug. Taking antidepressants for years, even decades, is an ongoing human experiment, which should not be taken lightly. Patients who may no longer need the drugs and want to try going off should be supported in doing so.

Trying to go off an antidepressant is a trial-and-error process. If necessary, the patient can always go back on the drug.

Notice that none of the criteria for establishing that a patient is ready to try going off an antidepressant is rigidly required or inflexible. I prefer the patient to meet at least criteria 1 and 2 but there are exceptions to the rule. For example, severe side effects like intolerable nausea, psychotic reactions, manic-like reactions, paranoia, hostility, aggression, or becoming suicidal may necessitate going off an antidepressant even when none of the other criteria are met.

After considering the above criteria, a patient may decide not to try going off his antidepressant, at least not yet. Or, he may decide with his doctor that all the signs are favorable to proceed to the next step in the 5-Step Antidepressant Tapering Program, making the first dosage reduction. Of course the above criteria are not an exhaustive list of factors to consider when evaluating whether to try going off one's antidepressant. Individual patients will have specific issues they need to address with their doctors.

Six Patients Whose Antidepressant Tapering Programs We Will Follow Closely

In the subsequent chapters of this book, we will examine six patients' antidepressant tapering programs in detail to thoroughly familiarize you with how to taper the drugs. Introduced in Chapter 6, the six patients are Claudia, Brent, Daria, Gary, Sarah, and Richard. All six patients tapered off 20 milligrams a day of Paxil. I chose six patients on Paxil because it is often used as the reference antidepressant when discussing antidepressant withdrawal since it causes the most frequent withdrawal reactions. I chose patients all tapering off the same dose to illustrate the wide range of withdrawal reactions seen in different patients.

Claudia

When I first met Claudia, she was a shy, waifish-looking woman in her late twenties with long blond hair down to her waist. Her watery green eyes had a perpetually startled, hypervigilant look. Claudia originally came to see me severely depressed, anxious, and suicidal. Initially, it was a mystery why the accomplished sixth grade teacher was so depressed. A new principal had recently taken the helm at her school and was making a number of changes. Still, Claudia took great pleasure in her teaching. The stress of a new administration hardly seemed adequate to account for her severe depression.

Claudia responded to a combination of psychotherapy and Paxil but really began her recovery only after she confided that her boyfriend of two years was verbally and physically abusive. Treatment with just an antidepressant would not have accomplished her divulging that she was in an abusive relationship and addressing the underlying cause of her depression. Claudia had a history of being abused by a stepfather and an earlier boyfriend. Part of why she was so devastated was that Claudia thought this boyfriend "was different." When he was abusive, Claudia became depressed to the point of being suicidal.

Claudia left the relationship with my support and encouragement. Her boyfriend pleaded with her to stay and even saw a therapist briefly himself, but Claudia did not feel he was truly motivated to change. In psychotherapy, Claudia came to understand how her early childhood abuse by her stepfather left her vulnerable to abusive men. From the beginning of their relationship, Claudia's ex-boyfriend had been impatient, demanding, controlling, and possessive. In retrospect, she saw these as "early warning signs" of his later abuse. Slowly, she became more assertive and less tolerant of ill-treatment in all aspects of her life, not just relationships. Gradually, her startled, hypervigilant stare softened into a more relaxed look as she became more self-assured.

Claudia also joined a support group for victims of domestic violence. The group helped her to feel less alone as she met other women who had been similarly scarred by childhood abuse. After two years in therapy and on Paxil, Claudia felt ready to try going off the drug. Claudia disliked the idea of taking medication if she no longer needed it and had also developed a side effect: On Paxil, Claudia had a tremor. Sometimes she was embarrassed by the tremor, when she reached for something in front of others or tried to demonstrate something using her hands. Especially since the tremor was a neurological side effect, she was concerned about the risks of staying on Paxil indefinitely.

Claudia met all six criteria for determining that she was ready to try going off an antidepressant. She was much improved; indeed, she had not been depressed, anxious, or suicidal for over a year and a half (criterion 1). The timing was favorable since Claudia waited to try going off the Paxil until she was in a stable period in her life without any unusual stress or crises (criterion 2). Claudia had grown a lot psychologically, having gained insight in psychotherapy and in the support group into how her childhood abuse had made her vulnerable to abusive relationships. She now expected better treatment from others and was a more assertive person (criterion 3). Claudia's circumstances changed dramatically when she left the abusive relationship that had made her depressed (criterion 4). She was motivated to go off the Paxil because she had a noticeable tremor on the drug (criterion 5). Claudia was concerned about the long-term risks of staying on a drug that was causing a neurological side effect. Claudia did not want to stay on an antidepressant "for life" if she no longer needed it (criterion 6).

Brent

Brent is a twenty-eight-year-old man who became severely depressed after losing his job as a website designer and programmer when the dot com bubble burst. Brent found himself unemployed in a slowing economy glutted with people who had skills like his. Just a few months earlier, Brent's wife had quit her job to stay at home with their firstborn, now three months old. Many new parents feel somewhat stressed by the responsibilities of parenthood at the same time that they feel overjoyed to have a child. But Brent also felt overwhelmed by his sudden unemployment and became severely depressed.

Fortunately, Brent responded well to the combination of psychotherapy and 20 milligrams a day of Paxil. It turned out Brent's father had been an alcoholic who abandoned the family. When Brent lost his job he felt "terrified" of not being able to meet his responsibilities to his wife and son, just like his father. As he pieced together how his past had compounded his anxieties about being unemployed and a new father, Brent felt better able to cope with his situation. Once he began to feel better, Brent mounted a job search, tirelessly applying and interviewing for positions. He persevered through many rejections before finally landing a highly competitive position managing a team of computer programmers. On the new job, Brent coped well with a steep learning curve. Once he settled in and felt secure on the job, Brent wanted to try going off the Paxil after a year on the drug. He had developed sexual side effects: he was having delayed ejaculation, which made it difficult for him to climax during sex.

Brent met five of the six criteria for determining that he was ready to try going off his antidepressant. His condition was much improved since he had not been depressed for almost a year (criterion 1). The timing was favorable, since Brent had waited until he settled into his new job before trying to go off his antidepressant (criterion 2). He had grown psychologically, having learned in psychotherapy how losing his job soon after his son was born triggered painful memories of his father being unable to support his family (criterion 3). His circumstances had changed now that Brent was thriving at a new job (criterion 4). Brent wanted to go off Paxil because of sexual side effects (criterion 5).

If Brent had felt he still needed to be on an antidepressant—because he was still depressed, his circumstances had not changed enough, the timing was not favorable, or he just did not feel ready to try going off his antidepressant—we could have switched him to another antidepressant in a different class less likely to cause sexual side effects. Since the new antidepressant would not be in the same class and would therefore not protect against Paxil withdrawal, Brent would have still needed to taper off the Paxil.

Daria

Daria was a twenty-year-old black woman and a sophomore at Harvard College when her mother died of emphysema and congestive heart failure. Daria had been quite stoical throughout her mother's long illness and death. But six months later when she moved home to Chicago for the summer, she became acutely anxious that she herself had a heart condition. Daria was convinced that aches and pains she felt in her chest were a sign of potentially fatal heart disease. Her anxieties were not allayed by multiple diagnostic tests that all showed her heart was perfectly normal. When she returned to Boston in the fall, it quickly became apparent that she might have to take a leave of absence from school because her anxieties were making it so difficult for her to function. At this point, Daria was referred to me.

A lively, engaging young woman, Daria has penetrating brown eyes, soft dark skin, and cornrows in her hair with colorful beads. When I met Daria, I thought that she should perhaps take a semester off from college to deal with her grief over her mother's illness and death. Daria's concerns about having a heart condition were psychosomatic, converting her unresolved grief into an obsessive preoccupation with having a bodily illness. Indeed, her concern about having heart disease echoed her mother dying of heart failure. Of course, psychologically speaking Daria did have a broken heart: she needed to grieve her mother.

Daria was adamant that she did not want to drop out of school, insisting that "would only make things worse." Instead, she wanted to see if intensive psychotherapy, twice a week, and medication could help her to stay in school and grieve her mother at the same time. I cautioned Daria that antidepressant medication, which can blunt people's emotions, might interfere with her normal grieving process. But she was insistent on trying an antidepressant because she wanted to avoid taking a leave of absence from school.

In fact, Daria did respond well to a combination of therapy and 20 milligrams a day of Paxil. In therapy she dealt with her sadness over her mother's death. At the same time, she became more aware of her anger over her mother's having been a chain smoker and generally taken poor care of her health, which led to her emphysema, heart failure, and early death. In complicated grief reactions, anger is often the emotion people are most conflicted over and torn up about. After making considerable progress in psychotherapy, and after ten months on Paxil, Daria wanted to try going off the drug at the end of the academic year because she was gaining weight on it. Daria had initially lost her appetite and five pounds when she went on Paxil. This side effect was more of a plus than a minus, as it is for many patients. However, as often happens, over time the antidepressant began to have the opposite effect on her appetite and weight: Daria not only put the five pounds back on, she gained an additional ten pounds. Daria wanted to try stopping the Paxil before she gained any more weight.

Daria met four of the six criteria for determining that she was ready to try going off her antidepressant. She had not been anxious or preoccupied with psychosomatic concerns about her health for more than six months (criterion 1). She decided in the spring of her junior year to try going off Paxil but waited for more favorable timing until after her exams were over to begin her tapering program (criterion 2). She had grown considerably in psychotherapy grieving her mother and coming to understand why she developed psychosomatic symptoms as a result of her earlier, unresolved grief (criterion 3). Daria wanted to go off Paxil because of significant weight gain (criterion 5).

Gary

Gary is a twenty-six-year-old Korean man who became depressed after a girlfriend of two years abruptly broke up with him. By the time I first saw him, Gary was so depressed he was in jeopardy of losing his job as a laboratory technician in a biotechnology company. Fashionably dressed, Gary cut a striking figure clothed all in black: shoes, slacks, T-shirt, sports jacket, and thick-rimmed glasses standing out against his pale skin and short-cropped black hair. Like many jilted men, Gary was making the mistake of aggressively trying to woo back his ex-girlfriend. In a vicious circle, Gary's imploring the ex-girlfriend to get back together again only made him less attractive to her and consequently made him feel worse about himself.

Gary responded well to a combination of psychotherapy and 20 milligrams a day of Paxil. Our initial focus in psychotherapy was scaling down his efforts to win back his ex-girlfriend. Through the psychotherapy, Gary gained a better understanding of why he reacted so strongly to the breakup, which resonated with his parents' sudden divorce when he was twelve years old. Gary gradually became angry with the ex-girlfriend over her treatment of him during the breakup, which helped him to get over her. Looking back on it, he began to feel he had been too passive in the relationship. Gary eventually began dating someone new, which led to what he felt was a healthier relationship. After nine months on Paxil, Gary wanted to try going off the drug. Although he had not had any side effects, Gary did not want to stay on an antidepressant if he no longer needed it. Like many patients, Gary was concerned about the long-term risks of staying on an antidepressant "indefinitely."

Gary met five of the six criteria for determining that he was ready to try going off his antidepressant. Gary was no longer depressed; he was in a relatively calm, stable period in his life (criteria 1 and 2). Through psychotherapy Gary had gained considerable insight into why he reacted so strongly, why he became so depressed when his ex-girlfriend broke up with him, and he was in a new, healthier relationship (criteria 3 and 4). Finally, Gary did not want to stay on Paxil indefinitely if he no longer needed it (criterion 6).

Sarah

Sarah had only been on Paxil for six months when she decided to try tapering off the drug. Sarah had an earth-mother look in flowing scarves and loose-fitting sweaters and blouses that draped over her calf-length skirts. She originally came to see me because of severe panic attacks and long-standing alcoholism. A thirty-three-year-old former secretary,

Sarah had been unemployed for a month because her alcoholism had made her so dysfunctional at work. Sarah started having panic attacks after she lost her job. She came into treatment quite scared by the setback in her life and motivated to turn around her drinking.

I could not use Valium-type drugs to treat Sarah's panic attacks because they act on the same receptors in the brain as alcohol and should not be prescribed to people with alcoholism. And, I could not start Sarah on Paxil for her anxiety until she stopped drinking, because the combination of antidepressants and alcohol can be quite dangerous. This increased Sarah's motivation to go to Alcoholics Anonymous, which I encouraged her to do. She used the program to successfully stop drinking without having to check into a hospital rehab program. Once she stopped drinking, I started Sarah on Paxil and also referred her to a ten-week cognitive-behavioral program for the panic attacks. The cognitive-behavioral skills she acquired helped Sarah manage her anxiety without resorting to alcohol. As is so often the case, Sarah's psychological treatment, AA, and the antidepressant were synergistic. After six months on the drug, Sarah was ready to try going off. I encouraged her to wait another three to six months because her sobriety and newfound progress were in a relatively early stage. But Sarah was insistent because she had severe sexual dysfunction on Paxil.

Sarah met four of the six criteria for determining that she was ready to try going off her antidepressant. Sarah was sober and no longer having panic attacks (criterion 1). She was in a relatively stable period in her life, not in any crisis (criterion 2). With the benefit of AA and cognitive therapy, she was better able to manage her sobriety and anxiety (criterion 3). Sarah was motivated to go off Paxil by severe sexual dysfunction (criterion 5). Note that Sarah did not meet criterion 4, a change in relevant circumstances. Obviously, her circumstances were much improved since she was sober and free of panic attacks. But the specific circumstance that led to Sarah's depression was being fired from her job. And, at the time that she decided to try tapering off her antidepressant, Sarah was still unemployed.

Richard

Richard was a forty-nine-year-old gay documentary film director who became depressed when a fire destroyed his studio and a film he was in the process of editing. At the time, Richard was on sabbatical from teaching in the film department at an arts college in Boston. He was living in Maine, finishing up a documentary on the fishing industry. The documentary had been accepted into a prestigious film festival and Richard felt devastated by the fire and the prospect of not being able to go to the festival. To turn the situation around, he would need to work feverishly to reshoot most of the film and quickly reedit it under intense deadline pressure. But his depression left Richard unable to get out of bed to work. Richard's family doctor started him on 20 milligrams a day of Paxil and he began seeing a therapist in an attempt to get back on his feet. He came out of his depression but not in time to complete the film for the festival.

Richard first came to see me a year later when he had moved back to Boston and was in the process of "putting his life back together." Richard hoped to be reinvited to the festival the following year, but had not yet heard from the committee. He was once again enjoying teaching and the support of his many close friends in Boston. Although no longer depressed, Richard had stayed on Paxil through his transition back to teaching. Once he settled back into his life in Boston, he wanted to try tapering off Paxil.

I was concerned that Richard might become depressed again if he was not reinvited to the film festival. But Richard assured me that through psychotherapy he had put the episode behind him. In retrospect, he realized he had cared too much about the honor and recognition the invitation to the film festival conferred on him. "A real artist can't care about that," Richard insisted. "I've always done films that I thought were important, not because they impressed other people. I surprised myself and let myself down when I realized how much I cared about the recognition. I want to go off the Paxil before I hear from the committee because I want to test myself, I want to prove to myself that if I don't get invited again I won't get depressed now."

In addition, Richard had developed a side effect of Paxil: He felt "fatigued" on the drug. Initially, when he went on Paxil Richard felt quite "caffeinated," almost to the point of being jittery. Richard did not mind this side effect, which helped to "jump start" him out of the depression and then gradually disappeared as Richard's brain and nervous system adapted to the drug. However, like many patients, over time Richard developed the opposite side effect: he felt fatigued or "sluggish." Because he no longer felt depressed but had this bothersome side effect, Richard wanted to try going off Paxil.

Richard met four of the six criteria for determining that he was ready to go off his antidepressant. He had not been depressed for almost a year (criterion 1). He had waited until after he transitioned back into teaching and living in Boston before deciding to try going off Paxil (criterion 2). Through psychotherapy he understood why he became depressed when the fire prevented him from going to the film festival (criterion 3). The fatigue that Paxil was causing Richard was part of his motivation to go off the drug (criterion 5). Note that Richard did not meet criterion 4, a change in relevant circumstances. A relevant change in circumstances would have been getting invited back to the film festival, which had not yet happened, or not getting invited and dealing well with the disappointment, that is, not getting depressed over it.

What if a patient had Richard's side effect, fatigue, but still felt he needed to be on an antidepressant because he was still depressed, the timing was not favorable, or he simply was not ready to try going off the antidepressant? We would address the fatigue in other ways. First, we would move the Paxil dose from the morning to the evening hoping that the fatigue would coincide with when he was sleeping. In some instances, that adjustment is enough to alleviate the side effect. If this did not provide enough relief, next we would have lowered the dose, hoping the fatigue would clear while the lower dose continued to work for him. If the fatigue continued to be a problem, we would switch to a different antidepressant. Whatever the side effect, one tries a variety of interventions to address it if the patient needs to remain on medication.

These six patients are representative of the patients I treat with antidepressants but may not be representative of the treatment you have received. Still, you may be ready to try going off your antidepressant. All six patients—Claudia, Brent, Daria, Gary, Sarah, and Richard—had moderate to severe symptoms of depression or anxiety that justified their going on medication. None of them had mild symptoms that would have been better treated without drugs. But some patients are put on antidepressants for mild, even trivial symptoms. This was the case for John who was discussed earlier in Chapter 3. John is the Harvard undergraduate who got into trouble with the law because he stole another student's backpack while in severe Paxil withdrawal. He was originally put on Paxil late in a year off from college when he told a doctor he was "apprehensive" about returning to school. In retrospect John probably never needed the antidepressant. Once John settled back in to school, the change in circumstances together with the fact that he was feeling fine justified his trying to go off the antidepressant. Many patients find themselves in John's position because today's antidepressants have been unnecessarily prescribed to people for mild, even trivial conditions.

All six patients were in psychotherapy with me in addition to being on medication. Claudia also joined a support group for women who have suffered domestic violence while Sarah joined AA and enrolled in a ten-week, cognitive-behavioral program for patients with panic attacks. So, all of them had psychological treatment in addition to treatment with an antidepressant. But many patients on antidepressants have not had psychological treatment, because their health plans did not offer or pay for much in the way of such treatment. This was true for John who would have been better served by short-term psychotherapy to address his apprehension about returning to school instead of being put on Paxil, if any treatment was needed at all. Diana, whose case was discussed in Chapter 1, is another example. Diana was treated by her doctor with Zoloft and did not receive supportive psychotherapy after her son Jason was severely injured in a car accident and needed multiple surgeries. Still, both John and Diana reached a point where they were feeling fine and their circumstances had changed enough (John was back in school and Diana's son was back to normal) so they felt ready to try going off their antidepressant without psychotherapy. You may feel the same way. Or, you may feel that you would like some psychological treatment, such as a ten-week cognitive-behavioral program to learn skills for managing anxiety, in preparation for going off the drug.

Whatever combination of criteria you meet and whatever special circumstances you have, the decision to try tapering off an antidepressant is ultimately yours. The decision needs to be well informed and carefully thought out together with your doctor. If your doctor feels unable to help you with the decision, you can always seek a second opinion. Of course, the decision to try tapering off an antidepressant is trial and error. You can always pause in the middle of a tapering program if you develop doubts about proceeding. And you can always go back on the antidepressant if you feel the need at a later date. Once you have decided to go ahead with tapering your antidepressant, the next step is making the initial dosage reduction.

8

Step 2: Making the Initial Dosage Reduction

You have probably already found your initial recommended dosage reduction in Table 6.2 "Recommended Tapering Programs for Today's Popular Antidepressants" (see page 93). However, do not make the reduction yet, without consulting with your doctor and reading this chapter and, indeed, the rest of the book, because there are exceptions to the rule and you need to understand how the 5-Step Antidepressant Tapering Program works in its entirety before starting a taper.

The initial dosage reduction is somewhat trial and error because you do not know what kind of withdrawal reaction you are going to have. The suggested initial dosage reductions in Table 6.2 are based on experience with many patients and are carefully chosen to be reasonable in size and to result in mild withdrawal reactions or no withdrawal reactions at all in the majority of patients. The initial dosage reduction for a particular patient is based on the following factors:

- The particular antidepressant the patient is taking
- How long the patient has been on the drug
- The patient's dose
- The patient's prior history, if any, of withdrawal reactions

Each of these factors is discussed below.

The Particular Antidepressant

Notice in Table 6.2 (page 93) that antidepressants come in pills of different doses. Different antidepressants are prescribed in 10-, 20-, 25-, 50-, 75-, or 100-milligram increments. So, the particular antidepressant influences what size dosage reductions you will be making as you go through the tapering program. A Paxil taper may go from a daily dose of 40 milligrams to 20 to 10 to 7.5 to 5 to 2.5 to 0, at monthly intervals. By contrast, an Effexor taper may go from a daily dose of 300 milligrams to 225 to 150 to 75 to 37.5 to 18.75 to 0 at monthly intervals.

How Long the Patient Has Been on the Drug

Almost all patients who have been on antidepressants for more than a month should use a tapering program when they are ready to try going off the drugs. The few exceptions are patients who have been on low doses for a couple of months or more. These are the lowest doses listed in Table 6.2, like 10 milligrams a day of Paxil, which do not need to be tapered, but instead can just be stopped. Still, many patients are on low doses precisely because they are exquisitely sensitive to drug side effects. So they may find they need to taper after all despite being on relatively low doses. One other exception is patients on 20 milligrams a day or less of Prozac who usually do not need to taper off, as seen in Table 6.2. But at higher Prozac doses, patients should taper off the drug.

Patients who have been on an antidepressant less than a month typically do not need to taper the drug. Since, in just one month, the brain has usually not yet fully adapted to living with the antidepressant, it does not need extra time to readjust to living without the drug. This assumes the dose was not rapidly escalated in the initial month the patient was on the drug. At the end of the first month, most of my patients are still only on the recommended starting dose of an antidepressant, for example 20 milligrams a day of Paxil. If I have put the patient up to 40 milligrams a day within the first month and we then need to stop it for some reason, I probably would put the dose back down to 20 milligrams a day and wait a week or two to see if the patient had any withdrawal symptoms before having him stop the drug altogether.

The Patient's Dose

Of course, the higher the starting dose of an antidepressant, the longer the taper will take. That is, for a given patient, it takes longer to taper off of 60 milligrams a day of Paxil than 20 milligrams a day.

Patients on higher doses typically make larger milligram size reductions, but, at the same time, smaller percentage size reductions than patients on lower doses, as seen in Table 6.2 (page 93). A patient taking 60 milligrams a day of Paxil would try going down to 40 milligrams a day, a 20-milligram drop that is also a 33 percent reduction. By contrast, a patient taking 20 milligrams a day would try going down to 10 milligrams a day, a 50 percent reduction. Even though for the patient on 60 milligrams a day the first reduction is a larger milligram size, it is a smaller percentage size and, in the long run, the patient has more reductions to make to complete the taper.

The Patient's Prior History of Withdrawal Reactions

The patient's past history of withdrawal symptoms is an important variable in selecting an initial dosage reduction. Occasionally, this is the patient's second or third time on Paxil and she can recount in detail her prior experience with stopping or tapering the drug. More commonly, the patient's only experience of withdrawal symptoms has been when she forgot to take her antidepressant for one or more days. Patients often do not remember these experiences until specifically asked about them.

Before one can ask patients if they have ever had an antidepressant withdrawal reaction, one needs to be sure they know what the symptoms of antidepressant withdrawal are. The patient and doctor should review the symptoms found in Table 8.1 "Daily Checklist of Antidepressant Withdrawal Symptoms." The symptom checklist can also be found in Appendix 1. The checklist is described in greater detail in the next chapter since it is primarily an instrument used for monitoring withdrawal symptoms after a dosage reduction.

The patient should have her own copy of the checklist. The doctor and patient should familiarize themselves with all the antidepressant withdrawal symptoms because some of the less common ones, like suicidal thoughts or impulses, can be dangerous. At the same time, they

Table 8.1 DAILY CHECKLIST OF ANTIDEPRESSANT WITHDRAWAL SYMPTOMS

The 5-Step Antidepressant Tapering Program

Name: _____ Antidepressant: _____

Day: _____ (1, 2, 3, etc. since last dosage reduction) Date: _____ Day of week: _____

Dose prior to this reduction: _____ mg/day   New dose: _____ mg/day

PSYCHIATRIC SYMPTOMS	✔	MEDICAL SYMPTOMS	✔
That Mimic Depression		*That Mimic the Flu*	
1. Crying spells		29. Flu-like aches and pains	
2. Worsened mood		30. Fever	
3. Low energy (fatigue, lethargy, malaise)		31. Sweats	
4. Trouble concentrating		32. Chills	
5. Insomnia or trouble sleeping		33. Runny nose	
6. Change in appetite		34. Sore eyes	
7. Suicidal thoughts			
8. Suicide attempts		*That Mimic Gastroenteritis*	
		35. Nausea	
That Mimic Anxiety Disorders		36. Vomiting	
9. Anxious, nervous, tense		37. Diarrhea	
10. Panic attacks (racing heart, breathless)		38. Abdominal pain or cramps	
11. Chest pain		39. Stomach bloating	
12. Trembling, jittery, or shaking			
		Dizziness	
Irritability and Aggression		40. Disequilibrium	
13. Irritability		41. Spinning, swaying, lightheaded	
14. Agitation (restlessness, hyperactivity)		42. Hung over or waterlogged feeling	
15. Impulsivity		43. Unsteady gait, poor coordination	
16. Aggressiveness		44. Motion sickness	
17. Self-harm			
18. Homicidal thoughts or urges		*Headache*	
		45. Headache	
Confusion and Memory Problems			
19. Confusion or cognitive difficulties		*Tremor*	
20. Memory problems or forgetfulness		46. Tremor	
Mood Swings		*Sensory Abnormalities*	
21. Elevated mood (feeling high)		47. Numbness, burning, or tingling	
22. Mood swings		48. Electric zap–like sensations in the brain	
23. Manic-like reactions		49. Electric shock–like sensations in the body	
		50. Abnormal visual sensations	
Hallucinations		51. Ringing or other noises in the ears	
24. Auditory hallucinations		52. Abnormal smells or tastes	
25. Visual hallucinations			
		Other	
Dissociation		53. Drooling or excessive saliva	
26. Feeling detached or unreal		54. Slurred speech	
		55. Blurred vision	
Other		56. Muscle cramps, stiffness, twitches	
27. Excessive or intense dreaming		57. Feeling of restless legs	
28. Nightmares		58. Uncontrollable twitching of mouth	

Global assessment of severity of withdrawal symptoms for the day

None	Mild			Moderate				Severe		
0	1	2	3	4	5	6	7	8	9	10
✔										

should be aware that the most common symptoms of antidepressant withdrawal are: anxiety, crying spells, fatigue, insomnia, irritability, dizziness, flu-like aches and pains, nausea, vomiting, headaches, tremors, and sensory abnormalities such as burning, tingling, or electric shock–like sensations.

Once the patient is familiar with the spectrum of symptoms, the following points need to be reviewed systematically to establish whether or not the patient has experienced withdrawal symptoms:

1. Have you deliberately *gone off* this or any other antidepressant in the past and experienced withdrawal symptoms?
2. Have you ever deliberately *lowered the dose* of an antidepressant and experienced withdrawal symptoms?
3. Have you *accidentally forgotten* to take an antidepressant and experienced withdrawal symptoms?
4. Have you ever *traveled out of town* on vacation or for work, *forgotten* to pack your antidepressant, and experienced withdrawal symptoms?

If the answer is "Yes" to any of the above, then for each incident ask the following:

5. What withdrawal symptoms did you have?
6. What was your dose before and after the reduction?
7. How many days after you reduced the dose or stopped the drug did the symptoms appear?
8. How many days did it take for the symptoms to peak?
9. How long did the symptoms last?
10. How severe were the symptoms?
11. Did you stop the antidepressant or lower the dose under the supervision of a doctor?
12. At any point were you unable to function at your normal level because of withdrawal symptoms?
13. Did you have to resume taking the antidepressant or put the dose back up because the withdrawal symptoms were so bad?

The goal of asking these questions is to get as clear a picture as possible of the pattern of a patient's antidepressant withdrawal reactions. The information is useful in predicting what symptoms the patient may experience now as she begins to taper the drug. All of the questions should be asked in detail because many patients forget episodes of antidepressant withdrawal unless asked specifically, as illustrated in the sample dialogue below:

DOCTOR: Have you deliberately gone off your Paxil or any other anti-depressant in the past and experienced withdrawal symptoms?

PATIENT: No. I've been on Paxil for two years and never tried to go off it before.

DOCTOR: Have you deliberately lowered the dose and experienced withdrawal symptoms?

PATIENT: No. I was originally put on 20 milligrams a day of Paxil. A month later I was increased to 40 milligrams a day, the dose I've been on ever since. I've never gone down on the dose.

DOCTOR: Have you accidentally forgotten to take Paxil and experi-enced withdrawal symptoms?

PATIENT: No. I take it faithfully.

DOCTOR: Have you ever traveled out of town for vacation or work, forgotten to pack your Paxil, and experienced withdrawal symptoms?

PATIENT: Oh, yes . . . now that you mention it. As a matter of fact, that's happened to me twice. Once I went on a business trip to New York for three days. The other time I went on a three-day weekend to Cape Cod. [Note that the patient answered "No" to three quite specific questions but had, in fact, experienced withdrawal which he only re-called on the fourth, detailed question.]

DOCTOR: What withdrawal symptoms did you have?

PATIENT: Both times I got a splitting headache. The headache was really excruciating. Like nothing I'd ever had before.

DOCTOR: Did you have any other withdrawal symptoms?

PATIENT: I don't think so.

DOCTOR: (asking in some detail about common psychiatric symptoms of withdrawal): Any anxiety, tearfulness, fatigue, insomnia, or irritabil-ity?

PATIENT: I felt anxious and fragile. I had to cancel my last business meeting in New York and we had to leave the Cape early because I couldn't take it anymore. [Note that the patient had forgotten the other symptoms, which were less memorable to him, until asked specifically.]

DOCTOR: (asking in some detail about common medical symptoms of withdrawal): How about dizziness, flu-like aches and pains, nausea, burning, tingling, or electric shock–like sensations?

PATIENT: I was dizzy. I remember when we were leaving the Cape, I couldn't carry my suitcase downstairs because I was feeling so dizzy. I had to ask my wife to carry it. I had to hold on to the handrail with one hand and use the other hand to brace myself against the wall. It was pretty bad. Now I remember, too, the car ride home was pretty awful because every time we hit a bump my head would be spinning. [Again, the patient had forgotten the dizziness until specifically asked about it.]

DOCTOR: (indicating the checklist of antidepressant withdrawal symptoms): Did you have any of these other withdrawal symptoms?

PATIENT: (after reviewing the checklist): No. I think that was it.

DOCTOR: You had been on 40 milligrams a day and you took none for three days?

PATIENT: That's right.

DOCTOR: How many days after you stopped the drug did the withdrawal symptoms appear?

PATIENT: We went to the Cape on Friday night and I woke up with the headache, dizziness, and anxiety on Sunday morning.

DOCTOR: So, on day two.

PATIENT: Correct.

DOCTOR: How long did the withdrawal symptoms last?

PATIENT: We were supposed to leave the Cape on Monday night, but we drove up midday because I couldn't take it any more. I knew it was the Paxil because the same thing had happened on the business trip to New York. I took the Paxil when I got home and the headache, dizziness, and anxiety started to go away in a few hours.

DOCTOR: How severe were the withdrawal symptoms?

PATIENT: They were pretty severe. I wouldn't have been able to go to work the next day if I hadn't restarted the Paxil.

Many patients will recall having had withdrawal symptoms but not remember the exact details of their onset, peak, and resolution, which is fine. The doctor is just trying to collect as much information as possible, as illustrated in the following sample dialogue.

DOCTOR: Have you deliberately gone off your antidepressant in the past and experienced withdrawal symptoms?

PATIENT: I tried to go off Paxil a year ago when I was living in Chicago and I couldn't get off because the withdrawal symptoms were so severe.

DOCTOR: What withdrawal symptoms did you have?

PATIENT: I couldn't get out of bed I was so dizzy. I was nauseous and throwing up. I couldn't stop crying. I was having nightmares that someone was chasing me with a gun. I missed three days of work and then finally went back up on the Paxil.

DOCTOR: You had only lowered the dose? You hadn't gone off the Paxil completely?

PATIENT: I'd gone down to 15 milligrams a day.

DOCTOR: From 20 milligrams a day?

PATIENT: Yes.

DOCTOR: Did you have any anxiety, fatigue, insomnia, or irritability?

PATIENT: No.

DOCTOR: How about flu-like aches and pains, tremors, headaches, sweating, burning, tingling, or electric shock–like sensations?

PATIENT: No. The dizziness, nausea, and vomiting were enough!

DOCTOR: How many days after you lowered the dose did the withdrawal symptoms appear?

PATIENT: I don't remember exactly. The symptoms started within a few days and it was a week later that I was bedridden.

DOCTOR: You went back up on the dose after a week?

PATIENT: Roughly.

DOCTOR: How many days did it take for the withdrawal symptoms to peak?

PATIENT: I don't think they had peaked. I felt so terrible that maybe they were at their peak. But I don't know because I went back up to 20 milligrams a day. I couldn't stand it.

DOCTOR: Did you lower the dose under the supervision of a doctor?

PATIENT: Yes, my family doctor agreed I probably didn't need Paxil anymore. He had told me to just go down by five milligrams. But, it didn't work.

DOCTOR: What did you do then?

PATIENT: Well, my doctor didn't seem to know what to do. He just put the dose back up and I've been on it ever since.

DOCTOR: That was a year ago?

PATIENT: Yes. Just this time last year. In the early fall.

DOCTOR: You had pretty severe withdrawal. We'll have to try smaller reductions like 2.5 milligrams a day.

PATIENT: I was already cutting the 10-milligram pills in half. Are there smaller pills?

DOCTOR: No. But you can cut the 10-milligram pills into quarters with a pill cutter.

PATIENT: Really?

DOCTOR: Or, you can use the liquid form of Paxil if we have to try even smaller doses.

PATIENT: I didn't know a liquid form existed.

DOCTOR: Yes. You can measure out quite tiny doses with a dropper.

These sample dialogues illustrate the importance of asking patients specific, detailed questions about antidepressant withdrawal symptoms.

Initial Dosage Reductions for Patients with Histories of Severe Withdrawal Reactions

The suggested initial dosage reductions in Table 6.2 (page 93) are guidelines only and should be modified based on the particular patient's history and circumstances. In particular, if a patient has a history of severe withdrawal reactions, then the initial dosage reduction needs to be based on the specific details of the patient's prior reactions. For example, if the patient has a history of developing incapacitating dizziness with 5 milligram reductions in his daily Paxil dose, then one would have to try even smaller reductions of 2.5 milligrams or less. If the patient does not recall the exact milligram size of an earlier attempt to reduce his dose and his medical chart is not available, then one might try an initial dosage reduction that is half the size of the suggested initial dosage reduction in Table 6.2. If after this small initial dosage reduction the patient has little or no withdrawal reaction, then for the second dosage reduction one can try the larger, recommended dosage reduction.

The Six Patients Whose Antidepressant Tapering Program We Are Following in Detail

In the previous chapter, I introduced the six patients whose antidepressant tapering programs we are following in detail: Claudia, Richard, Sarah, Gary, Daria, and Brent. All six of these patients tapered off 20 milligrams a day of Paxil. All of them had been on the drug for more than a month and none of them had a history of severe withdrawal reactions. So, following the guidelines in Table 6.2, all six patients made the suggested initial dosage reduction, lowering their Paxil dose from 20 to 10 milligrams a day.

Initial Dosage Reductions for Children

Chapter 12 discusses tapering children off antidepressants. Young children are more vulnerable to antidepressant withdrawal reactions than adults, because they metabolize, or inactivate, antidepressants faster.[1] For children, the initial dosage reductions should be half the size of the suggested initial dosage reductions in Table 6.2 (page 93). If after this small initial dosage reduction the child or adolescent has little or no withdrawal reaction, then for the next dosage reduction one can try the larger, recommended dosage reduction.

Initial Dosage Reductions for Patients Not on Standard Doses

Table 6.2 suggests initial dosage reductions for patients on the standard doses of today's popular antidepressants. But some patients are on unusual doses, like 30 or 50 milligrams a day of Paxil. If you are on one of these unusual doses, for the initial dosage reduction, lower your dose to the closest standard dose in Table 6.2. A patient on 50 milligrams a day of Paxil would reduce the dose to 40 milligrams a day. A patient on 30 milligrams a day of Paxil would reduce the dose to 20 milligrams a day.

Deciding When to Make the Dosage Reduction

In addition to agreeing on the size of the initial dosage reduction, the patient and doctor should explicitly agree on when the patient will make the reduction. This may be the next day after the appointment. Or, if the patient has a big presentation coming up at work, it may be two weeks later. "When you feel ready, you can go down to 40 milligrams a day" is *not* the way to leave things. Instead, one agrees: "You'll stay on 60 milligrams a day through your last exam on Thursday and then you'll go down to 40 milligrams a day on Friday."

Making Sure the Patient Has Enough Medication

Typically, the patient needs a new prescription for the new dose of medication. Together, the doctor and patient need to do the math to ensure the patient will have enough pills of the correct sizes to last for about a month. Dosage reductions are made roughly once a month. If the patient develops withdrawal symptoms, they typically peak and subside within two to three weeks. After the symptoms completely clear, another one to two weeks should elapse for the patient to fully recover from the episode of withdrawal before making another reduction.

If the patient is reducing her Paxil dose from 40 to 20 milligrams a day and has 15 of the 40-milligram pills left, she does not need a new prescription. She can break those pills in half to last a month. On the other hand, if the patient does not have any 40-milligram pills left, then she needs a new prescription for 30 of the 20-milligram pills.

Sometimes the math gets complicated. Supposing a patient on 20 milligrams a day of Paxil is going to reduce the dose to 17.5 milligrams. She needs a new prescription for 10-milligram pills. Some of the 10-milligram pills she will cut in quarters to get 2.5-milligram pieces. Each day she will take a full 10-milligram pill, a 5-milligram piece, and a 2.5-milligram piece for a total of 17.5 milligrams. She needs a prescription for 55 of the 10-milligram pills. It is imperative that the patient has the right combination of pills so she does not become stranded in the middle of an episode of withdrawal.

The slow release versions of antidepressants—such as Paxil CR, Effexor XR, Wellbutrin SR, and Wellbutrin XL—should not be cut in half. The gel matrix of the pills is essential to their mechanism. The mechanism is destroyed if they are cut. Moreover, cutting makes them shatter and crumble. In general, the only slow release medications that can be cut are those that are scored, because the matrix exists intact on either side of the score. Paxil CR, Effexor XR, Wellbutrin SR, and Wellbutrin XL are not scored, and should not be cut. If it is necessary to cut pills, the regular version, not the slow release version should be prescribed. Note in Table 6.2 the recommended dosage reduction for patients on 150 milligrams of Wellbutrin XL, Wellbutrin SR, and Zyban is from 150 down to 75 milligrams. None of these slow release forms of Wellbutrin is available in 75-milligram pills. Instead, use the 75-milligram regular Wellbutrin pill.

As you reduce the dose of your antidepressant, you need to stay in close touch with your doctor to be sure you continue to follow the prescribing guidelines for the drug. For example, Wellbutrin needs to be dosed carefully to avoid an increased risk of seizures.[2] This applies all the time, not just when reducing the dose. Patients need to work closely with their doctors to be sure that, as they reduce the dose, they continue to take the remaining dose properly.

Pill Cutters

The smallest size Paxil pill available is 10 milligrams. To get 5-milligram doses or smaller, patients need to cut pills in half, quarters, and sometimes even eighths. Whenever a patient is going to cut pills into pieces, check to see if the pills are scored. The indentation inscribed across the middle of a scored pill makes it easier to cleanly break in half. Table 8.2 "Doses Available in Antidepressant Pills" is a handy reference to the pill sizes available in most pharmacies and also indicates which ones are scored. You may need to check with your local pharmacy to see exactly what pill sizes they carry. Since some of today's popular antidepressants are already generic and can therefore be manufactured by any pharma-

Table 8.2 DOSES AVAILABLE IN ANTIDEPRESSANT PILLS

Shaded cells indicate easier to cut, scored pills. Paxil CR, Effexor XR, Wellbutrin XL, and Wellbutrin SR should not be cut; switch to the regular release form instead. Check manufacturers' official guidelines for the most up-to-date changes in available pill sizes.

SSRIs						
Paxil	Paxil CR	Zoloft	Celexa	Lexapro	Luvox	Prozac
10 mg	12.5 mg	25 mg	10 mg	10 mg	25 mg	10 mg
20 mg	25 mg	50 mg	20 mg	20 mg	50 mg	20 mg
30 mg	37.5	100 mg	40 mg		100 mg	
40 mg						

Additional SSRIs			
Prozac Weekly	Sarafem (Prozac)	Symbyax (Prozac/Zyprexa)	Pexeva (Branded Generic Paxil)
90 mg	10 mg	25 mg/6 mg	10 mg
	20 mg	25 mg/12 mg	20 mg
		50 mg/6 mg	30 mg
		50 mg/12 mg	40 mg

SNRIs			
Effexor	Effexor XR	Cymbalta	Serzone
25 mg	37.5 mg	20 mg	50 mg
37.5 mg	75 mg	30 mg	100 mg
50 mg	150 mg	60 mg	150 mg
75 mg			200 mg
100 mg			250 mg

Other					
Remeron	Remeron SolTab	Wellbutrin	Wellbutrin XL	Wellbutrin SR	Zyban
15 mg	15 mg	75 mg	150 mg	100 mg	150 mg
30 mg	30 mg	100 mg	300 mg	150 mg	
45 mg	45 mg			200 mg	

ceutical company, different companies may make different pill sizes available.

If the pill size required is not scored or if the patient has to cut the pills into quarters, pharmacies sell inexpensive, guillotine-style pill cutters that improve accuracy and are very convenient. The pill cutters are much easier, safer, and more accurate than using knives. Even with the pill cutter, some pieces will fragment and be lost if the patient is cutting pills into quarters or eighths. This will be inevitable until pharmaceutical companies make smaller doses available to facilitate tapers. One should periodically check the official information available from pharmaceutical companies, since they are under pressure to bring out smaller pills to help patients taper off their drugs.

Prozac is available as a generic drug or as the more expensive, still-patented forms Prozac Weekly or Sarafem. Prozac Weekly is a delayed release capsule containing 90 milligrams of the drug to be taken once a week.[3] Eli Lilly marketed this patented once-a-week form of the drug when the patent on the original daily Prozac was expiring. Since Prozac Weekly averages about 13 milligrams a day of Prozac, I switch patients to 10 milligrams a day for a month to alleviate the bigger peaks and troughs of the weekly, 90-milligram dose. After a month on 10 milligrams a day, patients can usually stop taking Prozac altogether without difficulty. Still another drug, Symbyax, is a combination of Prozac and the antipsychotic Zyprexa (whose generic name is olanzapine). Symbyax contains 25 or 50 milligrams of Prozac with 6 or 12 milligrams of Zyprexa.

Sarafem is a patented, pink Prozac pill marketed specifically for premenstrual syndrome.[4] Available in 10- and 20-milligram doses, it is the same drug as the much less expensive, generic form of Prozac. Sarafem is either taken continuously or for two weeks of each month. Patients taking Sarafem should follow the recommended tapering program for Prozac in Table 6.2 (page 93). At doses of 20 milligrams a day or lower, most patients can stop the drug altogether without difficulty.

Remeron is available in generic form or as the more expensive, patented RemeronSolTab.[5] RemeronSolTab dissolves in the mouth for patients who have difficulty swallowing. RemeronSolTab is not widely prescribed. Patients on RemeronSolTab can follow the tapering schedule recommended for regular Remeron in Table 6.2.

Pexeva is a so-called "branded generic" close cousin of Paxil. The generic drug in both Paxil and Pexeva is paroxetine. But Paxil contains paroxetine hydrochloride whereas Pexeva contains paroxetine mesylate.

Table 8.3 ANTIDEPRESSANTS AVAILABLE IN LIQUID FORM

Five milliliters is approximately one teaspoonful. Different liquid preparations provide the medication in different doses. For example, one teaspoon of liquid Paxil contains 10 milligrams of the drug, while one teaspoon of Zoloft contains 100 milligrams of the drug. Tiny doses are achieved by using a dropper.

Paxil	Zoloft	Celexa	Lexapro	Prozac
10 mg / 5 ml	100 mg / 5 ml	10 mg / 5 ml	5 mg / 5 ml	20 mg / 5 ml

The difference is unimportant when it comes to tapering the drugs. Although Pexeva is available in this country, it is not well known to doctors. But the FDA included Pexeva in its 2004 warning on antidepressant-induced suicidality.

Liquid Forms of Antidepressants

Cutting pills into pieces smaller than quarters becomes difficult to do. Some antidepressants come in a liquid form, making it possible to use a dropper to more precisely measure out small doses. The liquid forms of antidepressants tend to be extraordinarily expensive, but they may be necessary to achieve tiny doses of antidepressants. Table 8.3, Antidepressants Available in Liquid Form, lists the antidepressants offering this option.

Some antidepressant pills are capsules, which contain a drug in a loose, granular form and cannot be cut in half. Dividing a capsule is difficult. One has to open the capsule, pour the granules on a tabletop, and divide them in half. Some patients pour the contents of a capsule into a glass of water or juice, stir the powder, and drink half the liquid to get half the dose. It is important to fully stir the liquid before taking the second half. Obviously with these methods it is difficult to achieve the kind of precision one would like when tapering antidepressants. Some patients who experience severe withdrawal reactions even resort to making dosage reductions by counting out the beads in the capsules and slowly reducing the number they swallow. Since the beads typically vary in size, even this method is not exactly precise. Unfortunately, there is no way around the lack of precision until pharmaceutical companies make pills available in smaller doses.

Preparing Patients to Monitor Withdrawal Symptoms and Scheduling Follow-Up Appointments

Between the time when the patient reduces his dose and the next appointment, he needs to begin monitoring any withdrawal symptoms he develops. The patient should be given a two to three week supply of the Daily Checklist of Antidepressant Withdrawal Symptoms (Appendix 1). The patient fills out a checklist each day until all of his withdrawal symptoms completely clear. He could also be given the Graph of an Antidepressant Withdrawal Reaction (Appendix 2) to plot his daily scores, if he wishes. Both of these instruments are discussed in detail in the next chapter since they are an integral part of monitoring withdrawal symptoms.

The purpose of the next appointment will be to evaluate and monitor any withdrawal symptoms the patient develops. "Call me in a week or two if you're having any withdrawal symptoms" is *not* the way to leave things. Rather, a specific follow-up appointment—day, date, and time—is scheduled. Make the next appointment for the time when withdrawal symptoms are likely to occur. This will vary with the specific drug. With one of the short-acting antidepressants (Paxil, Zoloft, Celexa, Lexapro, Luvox, Effexor, Cymbalta, Serzone, Remeron, and Wellbutrin), this means three to seven days after the patient makes the dosage reduction. With the long-acting antidepressant Prozac, this means two to three weeks. Of course, the patient is encouraged to call sooner if he has any concerns or questions, especially about severe or dangerous withdrawal reactions like incapacitating dizziness or suicidal thoughts.

9

Step 3: Monitoring Withdrawal Symptoms After a Dosage Reduction

Following a dosage reduction, the next step in an antidepressant tapering program is monitoring any withdrawal symptoms the patient experiences. This step requires one or more appointments depending on the severity of the patient's withdrawal reaction.

Daily Checklist of Antidepressant Withdrawal Symptoms

The most convenient and systematic way to monitor a patient's withdrawal reaction is the Daily Checklist of Antidepressant Withdrawal Symptoms, Table 8.1 (page 119). The checklist is reproduced at the back of the book as Appendix 1. You can make Xerox copies of the checklist from the Appendix or, for convenience, print copies off the web at www.antidepressantsolution.com.

Systematically reviewing all the potential symptoms of antidepressant withdrawal is crucial to accurately diagnosing withdrawal reactions. Research has consistently shown that failing to be systematic leads to underdiagnosis of withdrawal reactions.[1] If the Checklist of Antidepressant Withdrawal Symptoms is not used, then the patient must be asked about each one of the antidepressant withdrawal symptoms. Since this can be a tedious task for both doctor and patient, the checklist provides a convenient alternative.

Each day the patient starts a new checklist by recording her name and antidepressant at the top, as seen in Table 9.1, an example of a completed checklist. The particular "day" is recorded, based on the number of days since the dosage reduction was made. Day 1 is the day of the dosage reduction. Patients usually do not get withdrawal symptoms the first day. An exception is patients on Effexor or Effexor XR who lower the dose too abruptly. Day 2 is the next day after the dosage reduction, and so on. As one monitors withdrawal reactions, one thinks in terms of day 1, 2, 3, and so on since the last dosage reduction. After each dosage reduction, one starts over again with day 1, and so on. In order to keep track of the particular dosage reduction—since there will be subsequent reductions—the patient also records the previous and new dose of the antidepressant, as well as the date and day of the week.

Using the checklist, the patient checks off all symptoms that have developed since the dosage reduction. If the patient gets a headache on day 2 that lasts until day 8, she checks it off on the checklists for each of those days. If she then gets a tremor on day 5 that lasts until day 11, she checks it off on the checklists for each of those days. On the checklist, the psychiatric symptoms are separated from medical symptoms. Within these categories, the symptoms are further subdivided so that clusters of symptoms can be quickly recognized.

In published research on antidepressant withdrawal, symptoms that are preexisting before each dosage reduction but worsen in frequency or severity are also counted.[2] For example, if before going down on the dose the patient had a headache, which then dramatically worsened, peaked, and went away in the two to three weeks typical of withdrawal symptoms, the headache would be counted as a withdrawal symptom. In my work with patients, I prefer to rely on new symptoms for diagnosing antidepressant withdrawal reactions. In my experience, patients usually have more than enough new symptoms to accurately diagnose antidepressant withdrawal reactions without having to count the occasional preexisting symptom that became worse.

Most patients have clusters of symptoms that are readily identified as antidepressant withdrawal. If questions arise over whether the symptoms are due to another psychiatric or medical condition, record them on the checklist and then discuss them with your doctor. Together, you and your doctor can use the guidelines discussed in detail in Chapter 3 to dis-

Table 9.1 SAMPLE DAILY CHECKLIST OF ANTIDEPRESSANT WITHDRAWAL SYMPTOMS

The 5-Step Antidepressant Tapering Program

Name: _Daria_ Antidepressant: _Paxil_

Day: _5_ (1, 2, 3, etc. since last dosage reduction) Date: _____ Day of week: _____

Dose prior to this reduction: _20_ mg/day New dose: _10_ mg/day

PSYCHIATRIC SYMPTOMS	✓	MEDICAL SYMPTOMS	✓
That Mimic Depression		*That Mimic the Flu*	
1. Crying spells		29. Flu-like aches and pains	
2. Worsened mood	✓	30. Fever	
3. Low energy (fatigue, lethargy, malaise)		31. Sweats	
4. Trouble concentrating		32. Chills	
5. Insomnia or trouble sleeping		33. Runny nose	
6. Change in appetite		34. Sore eyes	
7. Suicidal thoughts			
8. Suicide attempts		*That Mimic Gastroenteritis*	
		35. Nausea	✓
That Mimic Anxiety Disorders		36. Vomiting	
9. Anxious, nervous, tense		37. Diarrhea	
10. Panic attacks (racing heart, breathless)		38. Abdominal pain or cramps	✓
11. Chest pain		39. Stomach bloating	✓
12. Trembling, jittery, or shaking			
		Dizziness	
Irritability and Aggression		40. Disequilibrium	
13. Irritability	✓	41. Spinning, swaying, lightheaded	
14. Agitation (restlessness, hyperactivity)		42. Hung over or waterlogged feeling	
15. Impulsivity		43. Unsteady gait, poor coordination	
16. Aggressiveness		44. Motion sickness	
17. Self-harm			
18. Homicidal thoughts or urges		*Headache*	
		45. Headache	
Confusion and Memory Problems			
19. Confusion or cognitive difficulties		*Tremor*	
20. Memory problems or forgetfulness		46. Tremor	
Mood Swings		*Sensory Abnormalities*	
21. Elevated mood (feeling high)		47. Numbness, burning, or tingling	
22. Mood swings		48. Electric zap–like sensations in the brain	
23. Manic-like reactions		49. Electric shock–like sensations in the body	
		50. Abnormal visual sensations	
Hallucinations		51. Ringing or other noises in the ears	
24. Auditory hallucinations		52. Abnormal smells or tastes	
25. Visual hallucinations			
		Other	
Dissociation		53. Drooling or excessive saliva	
26. Feeling detached or unreal		54. Slurred speech	
		55. Blurred vision	
Other		56. Muscle cramps, stiffness, twitches	
27. Excessive or intense dreaming		57. Feeling of restless legs	
28. Nightmares		58. Uncontrollable twitching of mouth	

Global assessment of severity of withdrawal symptoms for the day

None	Mild			Moderate				Severe		
0	1	2	3	4	5	6	7	8	9	10
✓							✓			

tinguish withdrawal symptoms from depressive relapse and from other medical conditions.

How many symptoms constitute a withdrawal reaction? Researchers' views vary on how many symptoms are required to diagnose an antidepressant withdrawal reaction. Some researchers only require one symptom.[3] Others require two or more.[4] Researchers need black and white criteria so that everyone involved in the research project is consistent. But in office practice, doctors can be more flexible. I feel more comfortable diagnosing antidepressant withdrawal reactions when at least two symptoms are present. In my experience, patients rarely have just one withdrawal symptom. If after the first dosage reduction the patient has just one symptom, my interpretation of the symptom depends on how characteristic it is of withdrawal and whether there are other likely causes. For example, if the patient has classic antidepressant withdrawal-type dizziness with the sensation of water sloshing around in her head, worsening of the dizziness if she moves, and difficulty walking, especially climbing stairs, then I consider it a withdrawal symptom, because it is so typical of withdrawal and there are no other likely causes. If, on the other hand, the patient just has a headache, it could be a coincidence due to any number of other causes. So, I would wait to see if the headache recurs after subsequent dosage reductions. Sometimes the lone symptom recurs like clockwork after each reduction, in which case one feels confident that the symptom, although the only one, is the result of withdrawal. But with other patients, the lone symptom does not recur after subsequent dosage reductions and one assumes, in retrospect, that it was merely a coincidence.

Global Assessment of the Severity of Withdrawal Symptoms

Notice in Table 9.1 that in addition to checking off all the symptoms the patient experienced, she also made a global assessment of the severity of her symptoms for the day. The global assessment is based on the patient's worst symptoms and their effects on the patient's ability to function. The criteria for differentiating mild, moderate, and severe withdrawal reactions were discussed in Chapter 3.

Mild withdrawal symptoms are tolerated relatively comfortably and do not affect the patient's ability to function. Moderate withdrawal symptoms are uncomfortable and interfere with the patient's ability to function normally. Severe withdrawal symptoms include any serious or alarming symptoms (like suicidal thoughts or behavior), debilitating symptoms, or symptoms that force the patient to put the dose back up, restart the drug, or taper painstakingly slowly.

The global assessment is rated on a scale from zero to ten. The scale and criteria for the global assessment are summarized in Table 9.2. The absence of any withdrawal symptoms is scored zero. Mild withdrawal reactions are scored from one to three; moderate reactions from four to seven; and severe withdrawal reactions from eight to ten.

Following a dosage reduction, a number of possibilities exist:

- No withdrawal reaction, i.e. no withdrawal symptoms
- A mild withdrawal reaction
- A withdrawal reaction in the lower end of the moderate range
- A withdrawal reaction in the higher end of the moderate range
- A severe withdrawal reaction that is not quite bad enough to force the patient to go back up on the dose
- A severe withdrawal reaction that forces the patient to go back up on the dose

An example of each of these possibilities is discussed below, in the cases of the six patients whose antidepressant tapering programs we are following closely: Claudia, Richard, Sarah, Gary, Daria, and Brent. All were on 20 milligrams a day of Paxil when they entered their tapering programs and none had a prior history of withdrawal reactions. So, all of them made initial dosage reductions from 20 down to 10 milligrams a day. Paxil is often used as the reference drug when discussing antidepressant withdrawal and dependence, and I chose patients who all made the same dosage reduction to illustrate the wide range of withdrawal reactions possible in different patients in response to the same size dosage reduction. The same wide range of withdrawal reactions can occur with any of the recommended dosage reductions of any antidepressant.

Claudia's Lack of Any Antidepressant Withdrawal Reaction

Of the six patients whose antidepressant tapering programs we are examining in detail, Claudia had the easiest time. Claudia originally came to

Table 9.2 TEN-POINT RATING SCALE FOR THE GLOBAL
ASSESSMENT OF THE SEVERITY OF ANTIDEPRESSANT
WITHDRAWAL REACTIONS

SCORE	SEVERITY	CRITERIA
0	**No withdrawal reaction**	No withdrawal symptoms (from Symptom Checklist)
1–3	**Mild withdrawal reaction**	Presence of: • Withdrawal symptoms (from Symptom Checklist) that are tolerated relatively comfortably and do not affect one's ability to function normally
4–7	**Moderate withdrawal reaction**	Presence of: • Withdrawal symptoms (from Symptom Checklist) that are uncomfortable and negatively affect, even to a minimal degree, one's ability to think clearly and/or function normally
8–10	**Severe withdrawal reaction**	Presence of one or more debilitating or alarming withdrawal symptoms (from Symptom Checklist) that: • include suicidal thoughts, suicidal behavior, harm to oneself or others, hallucinations, or manic-like symptoms • make it impossible to function normally for all or part of the day • require putting the dose of the antidepressant back up after a dosage reduction • require restarting the antidepressant if it had been stopped altogether • require tapering the antidepressant painstakingly slowly by such small reductions that the tapering program will take more than four months

see me severely depressed, anxious, and suicidal because she was in an abusive relationship. With my support in psychotherapy, Claudia left the relationship. She later joined a support group for women who are victims of domestic violence. As she gained insight into how her history of childhood abuse made her vulnerable to abusive relationships, Claudia gradually became a more self-protective and self-confident person. After two years, Claudia wanted to try going off Paxil because she had a tremor on the drug and did not want to stay on it indefinitely if she no longer needed it.

When Claudia reduced her Paxil dose from 20 to 10 milligrams a day, she developed no withdrawal symptoms at all. For two weeks, each day she filled out her daily checklist. But the only checkmark she put on the pages denoted "0," or "None," on the global assessment of the severity of symptoms. Table 9.3 reproduces Claudia's Daily Symptom Checklist for day 4. Her checklists for the other days were identical to this one, since she did not have any withdrawal symptoms. Claudia's dosage reduction can be summarized: After reducing her Paxil from 20 to 10 milligrams a day, Claudia experienced no withdrawal symptoms; she had no noticeable withdrawal reaction.

Brent's Severe Antidepressant Withdrawal Reaction

While Claudia had the easiest time after her initial dosage reduction, Brent had the most difficult. Brent became severely depressed after losing his Internet programming job just months after his first child was born and his wife had decided to stay home with their baby. Brent used a combination of psychotherapy and Paxil to turn his depression around. After a grueling job search, landing a new job, and settling into it, Brent decided to try going off Paxil because he had developed sexual side effects.

After he reduced his Paxil dose from 20 to 10 milligrams a day, Brent had a severe withdrawal reaction that forced him to go back up to 20 milligrams a day. Table 9.4 reproduces all of Brent's daily checklists of antidepressant withdrawal symptoms. As you read the text, examine Brent's checklists carefully so you get a real feel for how the checklists work. On days 1 and 2, Brent had no withdrawal symptoms. However, on day 3 Brent developed anxiety, crying spells, malaise, dizziness, and flu-like

Table 9.3 CLAUDIA'S DAILY SYMPTOM CHECKLIST FOR DAY 4

Name: *Claudia*   Antidepressant: *Paxil*

Day: __4__ *(1, 2, 3, etc. since last dosage reduction)* Date: _____ Day of week: _____

Dose prior to this reduction: __20__ mg/day   New dose: __10__ mg/day

PSYCHIATRIC SYMPTOMS	✓	MEDICAL SYMPTOMS	✓
That Mimic Depression		*That Mimic the Flu*	
1. Crying spells		29. Flu-like aches and pains	
2. Worsened mood		30. Fever	
3. Low energy (fatigue, lethargy, malaise)		31. Sweats	
4. Trouble concentrating		32. Chills	
5. Insomnia or trouble sleeping		33. Runny nose	
6. Change in appetite		34. Sore eyes	
7. Suicidal thoughts			
8. Suicide attempts		*That Mimic Gastroenteritis*	
		35. Nausea	
That Mimic Anxiety Disorders		36. Vomiting	
9. Anxious, nervous, tense		37. Diarrhea	
10. Panic attacks (racing heart, breathless)		38. Abdominal pain or cramps	
11. Chest pain		39. Stomach bloating	
12. Trembling, jittery, or shaking			
		Dizziness	
Irritability and Aggression		40. Disequilibrium	
13. Irritability		41. Spinning, swaying, lightheaded	
14. Agitation (restlessness, hyperactivity)		42. Hung over or waterlogged feeling	
15. Impulsivity		43. Unsteady gait, poor coordination	
16. Aggressiveness		44. Motion sickness	
17. Self-harm			
18. Homicidal thoughts or urges		*Headache*	
		45. Headache	
Confusion and Memory Problems			
19. Confusion or cognitive difficulties		*Tremor*	
20. Memory problems or forgetfulness		46. Tremor	
Mood Swings		*Sensory Abnormalities*	
21. Elevated mood (feeling high)		47. Numbness, burning, or tingling	
22. Mood swings		48. Electric zap–like sensations in the brain	
23. Manic-like reactions		49. Electric shock–like sensations in the body	
		50. Abnormal visual sensations	
Hallucinations		51. Ringing or other noises in the ears	
24. Auditory hallucinations		52. Abnormal smells or tastes	
25. Visual hallucinations			
		Other	
Dissociation		53. Drooling or excessive saliva	
26. Feeling detached or unreal		54. Slurred speech	
		55. Blurred vision	
Other		56. Muscle cramps, stiffness, twitches	
27. Excessive or intense dreaming		57. Feeling of restless legs	
28. Nightmares		58. Uncontrollable twitching of mouth	

Global assessment of severity of withdrawal symptoms for the day

None		Mild			Moderate			Severe		
0	1	2	3	4	5	6	7	8	9	10
✓	✓									

     www.antidepressantsolution.com

Table 9.4 THE DAILY SYMPTOM CHECKLISTS OF BRENT'S SEVERE ANTIDEPRESSANT WITHDRAWAL REACTION

Daily Checklist of Antidepressant Withdrawal Symptoms

Name: Brent   Antidepressant: Paxil

Day: 1 *(1, 2, 3, etc. since last dosage reduction)* Date: _____ Day of week: _____

Dose prior to this reduction: 20 mg/day   New dose: 10 mg/day

PSYCHIATRIC SYMPTOMS	✓	MEDICAL SYMPTOMS	✓
That Mimic Depression		*That Mimic the Flu*	
1. Crying spells		29. Flu-like aches and pains	
2. Worsened mood		30. Fever	
3. Low energy (fatigue, lethargy, malaise)		31. Sweats	
4. Trouble concentrating		32. Chills	
5. Insomnia or trouble sleeping		33. Runny nose	
6. Change in appetite		34. Sore eyes	
7. Suicidal thoughts		*That Mimic Gastroenteritis*	
8. Suicide attempts		35. Nausea	
That Mimic Anxiety Disorders		36. Vomiting	
9. Anxious, nervous, tense		37. Diarrhea	
10. Panic attacks (racing heart, breathless)		38. Abdominal pain or cramps	
11. Chest pain		39. Stomach bloating	
12. Trembling, jittery, or shaking		*Dizziness*	
Irritability and Aggression		40. Disequilibrium	
13. Irritability		41. Spinning, swaying, lightheaded	
14. Agitation (restlessness, hyperactivity)		42. Hung over or waterlogged feeling	
15. Impulsivity		43. Unsteady gait, poor coordination	
16. Aggressiveness		44. Motion sickness	
17. Self-harm		*Headache*	
18. Homicidal thoughts or urges		45. Headache	
Confusion and Memory Problems		*Tremor*	
19. Confusion or cognitive difficulties		46. Tremor	
20. Memory problems or forgetfulness		*Sensory Abnormalities*	
Mood Swings		47. Numbness, burning, or tingling	
21. Elevated mood (feeling high)		48. Electric zap-like sensations in the brain	
22. Mood swings		49. Electric shock-like sensations in the body	
23. Manic-like reactions		50. Abnormal visual sensations	
Hallucinations		51. Ringing or other noises in the ears	
24. Auditory hallucinations		52. Abnormal smells or tastes	
25. Visual hallucinations		*Other*	
Dissociation		53. Drooling or excessive saliva	
26. Feeling detached or unreal		54. Slurred speech	
Other		55. Blurred vision	
27. Excessive or intense dreaming		56. Muscle cramps, stiffness, twitches	
28. Nightmares		57. Feeling of restless legs	
		58. Uncontrollable twitching of mouth	

Global assessment of severity of withdrawal symptoms for the day

None	Mild			Moderate				Severe		
0	1	2	3	4	5	6	7	8	9	10
✓	✓									

Daily Checklist of Antidepressant Withdrawal Symptoms

Name: Brent   Antidepressant: Paxil

Day: 2 *(1, 2, 3, etc. since last dosage reduction)* Date: _____ Day of week: 10

Dose prior to this reduction: 20 mg/day   New dose: 10 mg/day

PSYCHIATRIC SYMPTOMS	✓	MEDICAL SYMPTOMS	✓
That Mimic Depression		*That Mimic the Flu*	✓
1. Crying spells		29. Flu-like aches and pains	
2. Worsened mood		30. Fever	
3. Low energy (fatigue, lethargy, malaise)		31. Sweats	
4. Trouble concentrating		32. Chills	
5. Insomnia or trouble sleeping		33. Runny nose	
6. Change in appetite		34. Sore eyes	
7. Suicidal thoughts		*That Mimic Gastroenteritis*	
8. Suicide attempts		35. Nausea	
That Mimic Anxiety Disorders		36. Vomiting	
9. Anxious, nervous, tense		37. Diarrhea	
10. Panic attacks (racing heart, breathless)		38. Abdominal pain or cramps	
11. Chest pain		39. Stomach bloating	
12. Trembling, jittery, or shaking		*Dizziness*	
Irritability and Aggression		40. Disequilibrium	
13. Irritability		41. Spinning, swaying, lightheaded	
14. Agitation (restlessness, hyperactivity)		42. Hung over or waterlogged feeling	
15. Impulsivity		43. Unsteady gait, poor coordination	
16. Aggressiveness		44. Motion sickness	
17. Self-harm		*Headache*	
18. Homicidal thoughts or urges		45. Headache	
Confusion and Memory Problems		*Tremor*	
19. Confusion or cognitive difficulties		46. Tremor	
20. Memory problems or forgetfulness		*Sensory Abnormalities*	
Mood Swings		47. Numbness, burning, or tingling	
21. Elevated mood (feeling high)		48. Electric zap-like sensations in the brain	
22. Mood swings		49. Electric shock-like sensations in the body	
23. Manic-like reactions		50. Abnormal visual sensations	
Hallucinations		51. Ringing or other noises in the ears	
24. Auditory hallucinations		52. Abnormal smells or tastes	
25. Visual hallucinations		*Other*	
Dissociation		53. Drooling or excessive saliva	
26. Feeling detached or unreal		54. Slurred speech	
Other		55. Blurred vision	
27. Excessive or intense dreaming		56. Muscle cramps, stiffness, twitches	
28. Nightmares		57. Feeling of restless legs	
		58. Uncontrollable twitching of mouth	

Global assessment of severity of withdrawal symptoms for the day

None	Mild			Moderate				Severe		
0	1	2	3	4	5	6	7	8	9	10
✓	✓									

Table 9.4 THE DAILY SYMPTOM CHECKLISTS OF BRENT'S SEVERE ANTIDEPRESSANT WITHDRAWAL REACTION (CONTINUED)

Daily Checklist of Antidepressant Withdrawal Symptoms

Name: Brent   Antidepressant: Paxil

Day: 3 (1, 2, 3, etc. since last dosage reduction) Date: _____ Day of week: _____

Dose prior to this reduction: 20 mg/day   New dose: 10 mg/day

PSYCHIATRIC SYMPTOMS	✓	MEDICAL SYMPTOMS	✓
That Mimic Depression		*That Mimic the Flu*	
1. Crying spells		29. Flu-like aches and pains	
2. Worsened mood	✓	30. Fever	
3. Low energy (fatigue, lethargy, malaise)		31. Sweats	
4. Trouble concentrating		32. Chills	
5. Insomnia or trouble sleeping		33. Runny nose	
6. Change in appetite		34. Sore eyes	
7. Suicidal thoughts		*That Mimic Gastroenteritis*	
8. Suicide attempts		35. Nausea	
That Mimic Anxiety Disorders		36. Vomiting	
9. Anxious, nervous, tense		37. Diarrhea	✓
10. Panic attacks (racing heart, breathless)		38. Abdominal pain or cramps	
11. Chest pain		39. Stomach bloating	
12. Trembling, jittery, or shaking		*Dizziness*	
Irritability and Aggression		40. Disequilibrium	
13. Irritability		41. Spinning, swaying, lightheaded	✓
14. Agitation (restlessness, hyperactivity)		42. Hung over or waterlogged feeling	
15. Impulsivity		43. Unsteady gait, poor coordination	
16. Aggressiveness		44. Motion sickness	
17. Self-harm		*Headache*	
18. Homicidal thoughts or urges		45. Headache	
Confusion and Memory Problems		*Tremor*	
19. Confusion or cognitive difficulties		46. Tremor	
20. Memory problems or forgetfulness		*Sensory Abnormalities*	
Mood Swings		47. Numbness, burning, or tingling	
21. Elevated mood (feeling high)		48. Electric zap-like sensations in the brain	
22. Mood swings		49. Electric shock-like sensations in the body	
23. Manic-like reactions		50. Abnormal visual sensations	
Hallucinations		51. Ringing or other noises in the ears	
24. Auditory hallucinations		52. Abnormal smells or tastes	
25. Visual hallucinations		*Other*	
Dissociation		53. Drooling or excessive saliva	
26. Feeling detached or unreal		54. Slurred speech	
Other		55. Blurred vision	
27. Excessive or intense dreaming		56. Muscle cramps, stiffness, twitches	
28. Nightmares		57. Feeling of restless legs	
		58. Uncontrollable twitching of mouth	

Global assessment of severity of withdrawal symptoms for the day

None		Mild			Moderate			Severe		
0	1	2	3	4	5	6	7	8	9	10
✓										

Daily Checklist of Antidepressant Withdrawal Symptoms

Name: Brent   Antidepressant: Paxil

Day: 4 (1, 2, 3, etc. since last dosage reduction) Date: _____ Day of week: _____

Dose prior to this reduction: 20 mg/day   New dose: 10 mg/day

PSYCHIATRIC SYMPTOMS	✓	MEDICAL SYMPTOMS	✓
That Mimic Depression		*That Mimic the Flu*	
1. Crying spells		29. Flu-like aches and pains	
2. Worsened mood	✓	30. Fever	
3. Low energy (fatigue, lethargy, malaise)		31. Sweats	
4. Trouble concentrating		32. Chills	
5. Insomnia or trouble sleeping		33. Runny nose	
6. Change in appetite		34. Sore eyes	
7. Suicidal thoughts		*That Mimic Gastroenteritis*	
8. Suicide attempts		35. Nausea	
That Mimic Anxiety Disorders		36. Vomiting	
9. Anxious, nervous, tense		37. Diarrhea	✓
10. Panic attacks (racing heart, breathless)		38. Abdominal pain or cramps	
11. Chest pain		39. Stomach bloating	
12. Trembling, jittery, or shaking		*Dizziness*	
Irritability and Aggression		40. Disequilibrium	
13. Irritability		41. Spinning, swaying, lightheaded	✓
14. Agitation (restlessness, hyperactivity)		42. Hung over or waterlogged feeling	
15. Impulsivity		43. Unsteady gait, poor coordination	
16. Aggressiveness		44. Motion sickness	
17. Self-harm		*Headache*	
18. Homicidal thoughts or urges		45. Headache	
Confusion and Memory Problems		*Tremor*	
19. Confusion or cognitive difficulties		46. Tremor	
20. Memory problems or forgetfulness		*Sensory Abnormalities*	
Mood Swings		47. Numbness, burning, or tingling	
21. Elevated mood (feeling high)		48. Electric zap-like sensations in the brain	
22. Mood swings		49. Electric shock-like sensations in the body	
23. Manic-like reactions		50. Abnormal visual sensations	
Hallucinations		51. Ringing or other noises in the ears	
24. Auditory hallucinations		52. Abnormal smells or tastes	
25. Visual hallucinations		*Other*	
Dissociation		53. Drooling or excessive saliva	
26. Feeling detached or unreal		54. Slurred speech	
Other		55. Blurred vision	
27. Excessive or intense dreaming		56. Muscle cramps, stiffness, twitches	
28. Nightmares		57. Feeling of restless legs	
		58. Uncontrollable twitching of mouth	

Global assessment of severity of withdrawal symptoms for the day

None		Mild			Moderate			Severe		
0	1	2	3	4	5	6	7	8	9	10
							✓			

Table 9.4 THE DAILY SYMPTOM CHECKLISTS OF BRENT'S SEVERE ANTIDEPRESSANT WITHDRAWAL REACTION (CONTINUED)

Daily Checklist of Antidepressant Withdrawal Symptoms

Name: Brent   Antidepressant: Paxil

Day: 5 (1, 2, 3, etc. since last dosage reduction) Date: _____ Day of week: _____

Dose prior to this reduction: 20 mg/day   New dose: 10 mg/day

PSYCHIATRIC SYMPTOMS		MEDICAL SYMPTOMS	
That Mimic Depression		*That Mimic the Flu*	✓
1. Crying spells		29. Flu-like aches and pains	✓
2. Worsened mood		30. Fever	
3. Low energy (fatigue, lethargy, malaise)	✓	31. Sweats	✓
4. Trouble concentrating		32. Chills	✓
5. Insomnia or trouble sleeping	✓	33. Runny nose	✓
6. Change in appetite		34. Sore eyes	
7. Suicidal thoughts		*That Mimic Gastroenteritis*	
8. Suicide attempts		35. Nausea	
That Mimic Anxiety Disorders		36. Vomiting	
9. Anxious, nervous, tense	✓	37. Diarrhea	✓
10. Panic attacks (racing heart, breathless)		38. Abdominal pain or cramps	
11. Chest pain		39. Stomach bloating	
12. Trembling, jittery, or shaking		*Dizziness*	
Irritability and Aggression		40. Disequilibrium	
13. Irritability		41. Spinning, swaying, lightheaded	✓
14. Agitation (restlessness, hyperactivity)		42. Hung over or waterlogged feeling	
15. Impulsivity		43. Unsteady gait, poor coordination	
16. Aggressiveness		44. Motion sickness	
17. Self-harm		*Headache*	
18. Homicidal thoughts or urges		45. Headache	
Confusion and Memory Problems		*Tremor*	
19. Confusion or cognitive difficulties		46. Tremor	
20. Memory problems or forgetfulness		*Sensory Abnormalities*	
Mood Swings		47. Numbness, burning, or tingling	
21. Elevated mood (feeling high)		48. Electric zap-like sensations in the brain	
22. Mood swings		49. Electric shock-like sensations in the body	✓
23. Manic-like reactions		50. Abnormal visual sensations	
Hallucinations		51. Ringing or other noises in the ears	
24. Auditory hallucinations		52. Abnormal smells or tastes	
25. Visual hallucinations		*Other*	
Dissociation		53. Drooling or excessive saliva	
26. Feeling detached or unreal		54. Slurred speech	
Other		55. Blurred vision	
27. Excessive or intense dreaming		56. Muscle cramps, stiffness, twitches	
28. Nightmares		57. Feeling of restless legs	
		58. Uncontrollable twitching of mouth	

Global assessment of severity of withdrawal symptoms for the day

None	Mild			Moderate			Severe			
0	1	2	3	4	5	6	7	8	9	10
✓									✓	

← NEW ONSET (at items 2, 37)

← NEW ONSET (at item 49)

← SYMPTOMS NOW SEVERE

Daily Checklist of Antidepressant Withdrawal Symptoms

Name: Brent   Antidepressant: Paxil

Day: 6 (1, 2, 3, etc. since last dosage reduction) Date: _____ Day of week: 10

Dose prior to this reduction: 20 mg/day   New dose: 10 mg/day

PSYCHIATRIC SYMPTOMS		MEDICAL SYMPTOMS	✓
That Mimic Depression		*That Mimic the Flu*	✓
1. Crying spells		29. Flu-like aches and pains	✓
2. Worsened mood	✓	30. Fever	
3. Low energy (fatigue, lethargy, malaise)		31. Sweats	✓
4. Trouble concentrating		32. Chills	✓
5. Insomnia or trouble sleeping	✓	33. Runny nose	✓
6. Change in appetite		34. Sore eyes	
7. Suicidal thoughts		*That Mimic Gastroenteritis*	
8. Suicide attempts		35. Nausea	
That Mimic Anxiety Disorders		36. Vomiting	
9. Anxious, nervous, tense	✓	37. Diarrhea	✓
10. Panic attacks (racing heart, breathless)		38. Abdominal pain or cramps	
11. Chest pain		39. Stomach bloating	
12. Trembling, jittery, or shaking		*Dizziness*	
Irritability and Aggression		40. Disequilibrium	
13. Irritability	✓	41. Spinning, swaying, lightheaded	✓
14. Agitation (restlessness, hyperactivity)		42. Hung over or waterlogged feeling	
15. Impulsivity		43. Unsteady gait, poor coordination	
16. Aggressiveness		44. Motion sickness	
17. Self-harm		*Headache*	
18. Homicidal thoughts or urges		45. Headache	
Confusion and Memory Problems		*Tremor*	
19. Confusion or cognitive difficulties		46. Tremor	
20. Memory problems or forgetfulness		*Sensory Abnormalities*	
Mood Swings		47. Numbness, burning, or tingling	
21. Elevated mood (feeling high)		48. Electric zap-like sensations in the brain	
22. Mood swings		49. Electric shock-like sensations in the body	✓
23. Manic-like reactions		50. Abnormal visual sensations	
Hallucinations		51. Ringing or other noises in the ears	
24. Auditory hallucinations		52. Abnormal smells or tastes	
25. Visual hallucinations		*Other*	
Dissociation		53. Drooling or excessive saliva	
26. Feeling detached or unreal		54. Slurred speech	
Other		55. Blurred vision	
27. Excessive or intense dreaming		56. Muscle cramps, stiffness, twitches	
28. Nightmares		57. Feeling of restless legs	
		58. Uncontrollable twitching of mouth	

Global assessment of severity of withdrawal symptoms for the day

None	Mild			Moderate			Severe			
0	1	2	3	4	5	6	7	8	9	10
✓										✓

← SYMPTOMS CONTINUE TO WORSEN

Table 9.4 THE DAILY SYMPTOM CHECKLISTS OF BRENT'S SEVERE ANTIDEPRESSANT WITHDRAWAL REACTION (CONTINUED)

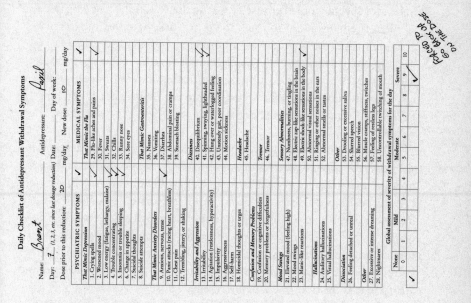

Daily Checklist of Antidepressant Withdrawal Symptoms

Name: Brent   Antidepressant: Paxil

Day: 7 (1, 2, 3, etc. since last dosage reduction) Date: ___ Day of week: ___

Dose prior to this reduction: 20 mg/day   New dose: 10 mg/day

PSYCHIATRIC SYMPTOMS

That Mimic Depression
1. Crying spells
2. Worsened mood
3. Low energy (fatigue, lethargy, malaise)
4. Trouble concentrating
5. Insomnia or trouble sleeping
6. Change in appetite
7. Suicidal thoughts
8. Suicide attempts

That Mimic Anxiety Disorders
9. Anxious, nervous, tense
10. Panic attacks (racing heart, breathless)
11. Chest pain
12. Trembling, jittery, or shaking

Irritability and Aggression
13. Irritability
14. Agitation (restlessness, hyperactivity)
15. Impulsivity
16. Aggressiveness
17. Self-harm
18. Homicidal thoughts or urges

Confusion and Memory Problems
19. Confusion or cognitive difficulties
20. Memory problems or forgetfulness

Mood Swings
21. Elevated mood (feeling high)
22. Mood swings
23. Manic-like reactions

Hallucinations
24. Auditory hallucinations
25. Visual hallucinations

Dissociation
26. Feeling detached or unreal

Other
27. Excessive or intense dreaming
28. Nightmares

MEDICAL SYMPTOMS

That Mimic the Flu
29. Flu-like aches and pains
30. Fever
31. Sweats
32. Chills
33. Runny nose
34. Sore eyes

That Mimic Gastroenteritis
35. Nausea
36. Vomiting
37. Diarrhea
38. Abdominal pain or cramps
39. Stomach bloating

Dizziness
40. Disequilibrium
41. Spinning, swaying, lightheaded
42. Hung over or waterlogged feeling
43. Unsteady gait, poor coordination
44. Motion sickness

Headache
45. Headache

Tremor
46. Tremor

Sensory Abnormalities
47. Numbness, burning, or tingling
48. Electric zap-like sensations in the brain
49. Electric shock-like sensations in the body
50. Abnormal visual sensations
51. Ringing or other noises in the ears
52. Abnormal smells or tastes

Other
53. Drooling or excessive saliva
54. Slurred speech
55. Blurred vision
56. Muscle cramps, stiffness, twitches
57. Feeling of restless legs
58. Uncontrollable twitching of mouth

Global assessment of severity of withdrawal symptoms for the day

None	Mild			Moderate				Severe		
0	1	2	3	4	5	6	7	8	9	10

(Forced to go back to old dose)

aches and pains. Although the psychiatric symptoms—the crying spells and anxiety—resembled Brent's original psychiatric condition, their timing and the simultaneous presence of characteristic medical symptoms of withdrawal clearly indicated he was having a withdrawal reaction. On day 3, Brent's global assessment of the severity of his symptoms was a 5, in the moderate range. But by the next day he felt considerably worse and rated the symptoms a 7, at the high end of the moderate range.

Brent and I met on day 5, as previously scheduled given the likely time course of Paxil withdrawal, to evaluate his withdrawal symptoms. Brent's dizziness was worsening; rooms seemed to him to be spinning and he had trouble walking up stairs. In addition, as seen on his checklist for day 5, he had four other new symptoms: Brent was having trouble concentrating after sleeping poorly the night before. Most disturbing to him, Brent had developed electric shock–like sensations up and down his legs and around his mouth. He rated his symptoms an 8, in the severe range, because the electric shock–like sensations were alarming to him and because he was unable to function at his normal level.

In our appointment, Brent said he wanted to persevere despite the severe symptoms. I knew from his earlier grueling job search that Brent could mobilize perseverance and determination. But the next day he had to leave work because the dizziness was so severe. At home, he had to lie in bed for several hours because he was so dizzy. On the morning of day 7, when Brent again felt too sick to go to work, he called me to say he "couldn't take" the withdrawal symptoms any longer and wanted to go back up on his Paxil dose to 20 milligrams a day. Brent was upset that he had to go back up on the dose but felt he "had no choice" since his symptoms had still not peaked and were intensifying. Within hours of taking a Paxil pill, Brent's symptoms began to improve and they were gone the next day.

When severe withdrawal symptoms force a patient to go back up on the dose, the patient resumes taking the dose he was on prior to the reduction. Brent therefore went back up to 20 milligrams a day. A patient in Brent's position does not go up to an intermediate dose, like 15 milligrams a day, because one cannot be sure that such a dose will be adequate. By the time a patient's withdrawal reaction is severe enough to force him to go back up on the dose, the patient is typically extremely uncomfortable and often debilitated, like Brent. At that point, one cannot afford to take the time to try an intermediate dose to see if it will be sufficient. Rather, one goes back up to the dose prior to the reduction, knowing that it will reliably clear up the withdrawal symptoms. One waits two weeks after all the withdrawal symptoms have cleared before trying a smaller dosage reduction.

Graphing an Antidepressant Withdrawal Reaction

Brent's daily assessments of the severity of his withdrawal symptoms are plotted in Figure 9.1, "Six Patients' Antidepressant Withdrawal Reactions." Figure 9.1 includes graphs of the antidepressant withdrawal reactions of all six patients whose antidepressant tapering programs we are following closely. Brent's graph can be found at the bottom of the second page of Figure 9.1.

A blank "Graph of an Antidepressant Withdrawal Reaction" can be found in Appendix 2 at the back of the book. Not all patients will want to fill out graphs of their antidepressant withdrawal reactions, but some will. The graph can provide a vivid picture of the pattern of a patient's withdrawal symptoms: their onset, peak, resolution, and severity. To be

Figure 9.1 SIX PATIENTS' ANTIDEPRESSANT WITHDRAWAL REACTIONS

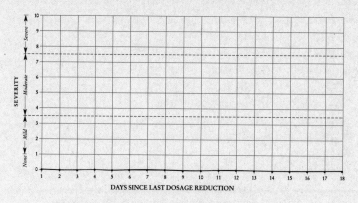

Claudia's Lack of Any Antidepressant Withdrawal Reaction

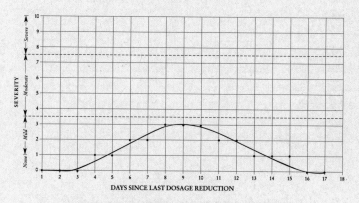

Richard's Mild Antidepressant Withdrawal Reaction

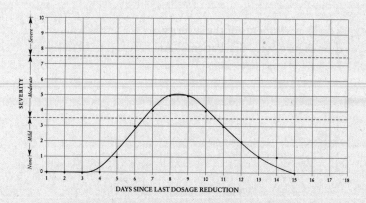

Sarah's Moderate Antidepressant Withdrawal Reaction

Figure 9.1 SIX PATIENTS' ANTIDEPRESSANT WITHDRAWAL REACTIONS (CONTINUED)

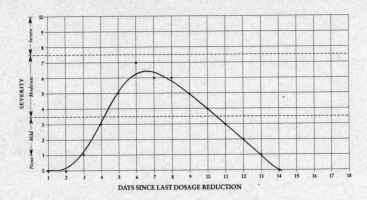

Gary's Moderate Antidepressant Withdrawal Reaction

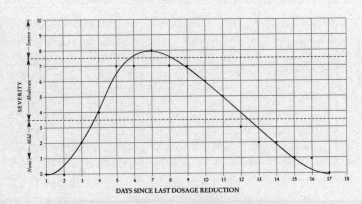

Daria's Severe Antidepressant Withdrawal Reaction

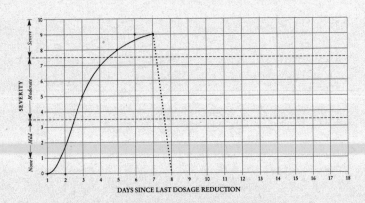

Brent's Severe Antidepressant Withdrawal Reaction

sure you understand how a graph is generated, review Brent's daily checklists in Table 9.4 (pages 140–143). At the bottom of each checklist, note Brent's daily global assessment of the severity of his symptoms and match it to the corresponding point on his graph in Figure 9.1: zero for days 1 and 2, five for day 3, seven for day 4, eight for day 5, and nine for days 6 and 7.

In Figure 9.1, one can see Brent's symptoms rise steeply into the severe range within days of lowering his Paxil dose to 10 milligrams a day. On day 7, when he went back up to 20 milligrams a day, his withdrawal symptoms disappeared within 24 hours as indicated by the dotted line.

While one monitors antidepressant withdrawal reactions, one also evaluates them. This becomes especially important for the next step in an antidepressant tapering program, Making Additional Dosage Reductions, discussed in Chapter 10. One chooses the size of the next dosage reduction based on the patient's reaction to the previous reduction. Obviously, no withdrawal reaction or mild withdrawal reactions are the most comfortable and, therefore, desirable for patients. Patients who have little or no withdrawal reaction can simply proceed with the next recommended dosage reduction for their particular antidepressant. Severe withdrawal reactions are unacceptable and not to be repeated. Patients who have moderate to severe withdrawal reactions cannot proceed with the next recommended dosage reduction. Instead, they make smaller dosage reductions, customizing them according to the guidelines in Chapter 10: Making Additional Dosage Reductions.

In the graphs in Figure 9.1, the horizontal, dashed lines separate the mild, moderate, and severe ranges. Clearly Brent's withdrawal reaction was well within the unacceptable, severe range. Notice that Brent's graph is at the opposite end of the spectrum from Claudia's at the top of the first page of Figure 9.1. Claudia's graph is a flat line because she had no symptoms, whereas Brent's is a steep curve that culminates in his having to go back up on the dose to suppress severe withdrawal symptoms.

The graphs shown in Figure 9.1 cover a two-and-a-half-week period. Some patients experience withdrawal symptoms that last longer.[5] Under these circumstances, one needs to modify the graph, use more than one, or prepare an alternative graph to accommodate a longer time period.

When a patient has to go back up on the dose like Brent because of severe withdrawal reactions, his doctor typically needs to give him a new prescription so he will not run out of medication on the higher dose. Brent's episode of withdrawal can be summarized: After reducing his

Paxil dose from 20 to 10 milligrams a day, Brent had seven days of severe withdrawal symptoms that resulted in his having to go back up on the dose to suppress an incapacitating withdrawal reaction. While Claudia's and Brent's withdrawal reactions represent the opposite ends of the spectrum, a range of possibilities exist in between, as seen in Richard's, Sarah's, Gary's, and Daria's reactions in Figure 9.1.

Richard's Mild Antidepressant Withdrawal Reaction

Like Claudia, Richard had a relatively easy time when he reduced his Paxil dose from 20 to 10 milligrams a day. Richard is the documentary film director who became depressed when his studio was destroyed by a fire, which prevented him from taking his documentary film about the Maine fishing industry to a prestigious film festival that he had been invited to. After more than a year on Paxil, Richard wanted to try tapering off of it, because he was no longer depressed and had developed the side effect of feeling "fatigued" and "sluggish" on the drug.

Richard's mild antidepressant withdrawal reaction after his initial dosage reduction is plotted in the second graph in Figure 9.1 (pages 145–146). When Richard reduced his Paxil dose, he had a mild withdrawal reaction. Although he developed dizziness, a "cotton wool feeling" in his head, blurred vision, and a tremor, Richard tolerated these symptoms relatively comfortably and they did not interfere with his ability to function normally. In Richard's graph, one can see his antidepressant withdrawal symptoms peak and wane without ever leaving the mild range. Richard's reaction can be summarized: After reducing his Paxil dose from 20 to 10 milligrams a day, Richard tolerated mild withdrawal symptoms relatively well for a little over two weeks.

When tapering antidepressants, one is aiming for reactions like Claudia's or Richard's, that is, mild withdrawal reactions or no withdrawal reaction at all. Because the dosage reductions in the 5-Step Antidepressant Tapering Program are of reasonable size and based on experience with many patients, the majority of patients will have little or no withdrawal reaction, like Claudia and Richard.

Sarah's Withdrawal Reaction in the Lower End of the Moderate Range

Sarah is the earth-mother office manager in flowing scarves who, after losing her job because of her alcoholism, became so anxious that she developed panic attacks, and therefore had a new motivation to overcome her addiction. She used a combination of psychotherapy, Alcoholics Anonymous, cognitive-behavioral skills, and Paxil to establish sobriety and overcome the panic attacks. Sarah insisted on going off Paxil after just six months because of sexual side effects.

When Sarah reduced her Paxil dose from 20 to 10 milligrams a day, she had a moderate reaction, consisting entirely of psychiatric symptoms: crying spells, feeling depressed, low energy, trouble sleeping, confusion, memory problems, and trouble concentrating. However, Sarah's symptoms remained moderate. In Figure 9.1 (page 145), one can see Sarah's symptoms start on day 5, peak in the lower end of the moderate range on days 8 and 9, and clear on day 15. Although Sarah only had psychiatric withdrawal symptoms, their characteristic time course clearly indicated they were an antidepressant withdrawal reaction. Sarah's reaction can be summarized: After reducing her Paxil dose from 20 to 10 milligrams a day, Sarah experienced two weeks of psychiatric withdrawal symptoms in the lower end of the moderate range.

Gary's Withdrawal Reaction in the Higher End of the Moderate Range

Gary is the biotech laboratory technician dressed in all black who became severely depressed when his girlfriend of two years abruptly broke up with him. Gary used a combination of psychotherapy and Paxil to overcome his depression. After nine months on the drug, Gary was no longer depressed and wanted to go off Paxil because he was concerned about the long-term risks of staying on it indefinitely.

When Gary reduced his Paxil dose from 20 to 10 milligrams a day, his withdrawal reaction consisted almost entirely of medical symptoms: dizziness, feeling like his head was "waterlogged," flu-like aches and pains, chills, and sweats. Gary also had abnormal visual sensations: he felt that his view was "randomly jumping" from side to side even when he

was sitting or standing perfectly still. Gary had one psychiatric withdrawal symptom: he became irritable with his coworkers and friends.
Since his symptoms were clearly affecting his work, he rated them in the
high moderate range.

In Figure 9.1 (page 145), one can see Gary's withdrawal symptoms
peak on day 6 and gradually resolve by day 14. Although Gary was able
to tolerate his withdrawal reaction, he did not find it acceptable, and he
wanted to make a smaller dosage reduction the next time. Gary's reaction
can be summarized: After reducing his Paxil dose from 20 to 10 milligrams a day, Gary experienced thirteen days of antidepressant withdrawal symptoms in the higher end of the moderate range.

Daria's Severe Withdrawal Reaction

Daria is the Harvard undergraduate whose mother died of emphysema
and congestive heart failure. After her mother's death, Daria developed a
debilitating psychosomatic fear that she, too, had a potentially fatal heart
condition and almost had to drop out of her sophomore year of college.
In ten months of psychotherapy, Daria began to work through her grief
over her mother's death and her anger that her mother, a life-long smoker,
had not taken better care of her health. With her psychosomatic concerns
behind her and doing well in school, Daria wanted to go off Paxil because
she was steadily gaining weight on the drug.

When Daria reduced her dose from 20 to 10 milligrams a day, she had
a severe withdrawal reaction: severe nausea, vomiting, abdominal pain,
depressed mood, and irritability. In Figure 9.1, one can see her symptoms
begin on day 3, peak on day 7, and resolve by day 17. If you compare
the graphs of Daria's and Brent's withdrawal reactions, you can see that
Brent's was slightly more severe, just enough to require increasing the
dose again. Of course, when Daria and I planned her next dosage reduction, we did not want to repeat such a severe withdrawal reaction, as
discussed in the next chapter. Daria's withdrawal reaction can be summarized: After reducing her Paxil dose from 20 to 10 milligrams a day, Daria
had sixteen days of severe symptoms which were not quite bad enough to
force her to go back up on the dose.

The Spectrum of Withdrawal Reactions

The graphs in Figure 9.1 (pages 145–146) summarize the antidepressant withdrawal reactions of Claudia, Richard, Sarah, Gary, Daria, and Brent. We will continue to follow these patients' progress in the next several chapters, looking at the ongoing course of their antidepressant tapering programs.

All six patients reduced their Paxil dose from 20 to 10 milligrams a day. Their graphs illustrate the wide range of withdrawal reactions in patients on the same antidepressant, making the same initial dosage reductions. There is no "normal," "average," or "typical" withdrawal reaction in response to a dosage reduction. The wide range of possibilities and the unpredictability of withdrawal reactions are reasons why one has to customize dosage reductions through a trial-and-error process.

Notice that once patients have been on antidepressants for more than about a month, there is no correlation between how long patients have been on antidepressants and how severe their withdrawal reactions are. Claudia had been on Paxil for two years—longer than any of the other patients—yet she had no withdrawal reaction following the same dosage reduction that the others made. Nor is there any correlation with the severity of the patient's original psychiatric condition. Here again, Claudia was in the worst shape coming into treatment; she was in an abusive relationship and suicidally depressed. But when she went off Paxil, Claudia had the easiest time lowering her dose.

When patients stop antidepressants cold turkey, 66 percent of patients stopping Paxil, 60 percent of patients stopping Zoloft, and 78 percent of patients stopping Effexor have withdrawal reactions.[6] What percent have mild versus moderate versus severe reactions? We do not have a definitive answer to this question; the research simply has not been done. Unfortunately, most doctors and patients are not attuned to the problem of antidepressant withdrawal reactions. As a result, patients can suffer high rates of withdrawal reactions, including severe withdrawal. However, following the guidelines of the 5-Step Antidepressant Tapering Program, in my experience most patients have no withdrawal reaction at all or mild withdrawal reactions that they tolerate comfortably. Few patients have withdrawal reactions that are so severe they are forced to go back up on the dose like Brent was. Even after subsequent dosage reductions, patients rarely have to put the dose back up, because subsequent reductions are further customized and adjusted based on the patients' initial withdrawal reactions.

The six patients in Figure 9.1 represent the spectrum of *severity* of antidepressant withdrawal reactions, ranging from no reaction to severe reactions that necessitate the patient going back up on the dose. While all the patients in Figure 9.1 reduced their daily Paxil dose from 20 down to 10 milligrams, the same range of possibilities exists with any recommended dosage reduction of any antidepressant. One could pick six other patients who had the same spectrum of reactions after lowering their daily dose from 40 down to 20 milligrams, or from 60 down to 40 milligrams, or from 10 down to 7.5 milligrams. The patients would have their own unique clusters of withdrawal symptoms, but these are the range of possibilities in terms of the *severity* of their reactions.

While Figure 9.1 covers the spectrum in terms of severity, it does not cover the range of possibilities in terms of the timing of antidepressant withdrawal reactions, that is, the onset, peak, and resolution of withdrawal symptoms. The graphs are typical of patients who develop withdrawal symptoms on about day 3 to 5, whose symptoms peak around day 7 to 10, and last no more than two to three weeks. But some patients develop antidepressant withdrawal symptoms even faster, on day 1 or day 2. Other patients do not develop symptoms until day 6 or later. Some patients' withdrawal symptoms last longer than three weeks. This also varies with the specific drug.

Antidepressant withdrawal reactions like those seen in the patients followed in this chapter and summarized in Figure 9.1 are typical only when patients are being carefully tapered off their drug. The "horror stories" one hears of much more severe withdrawal reactions or withdrawal reactions that last far longer are much more likely to occur when patients are not warned of antidepressant withdrawal and stop the drugs cold turkey, drop the dose precipitously, or taper off too quickly.

Scheduling Follow-up Appointments

This step in an Antidepressant Tapering Program—Step 3, Monitoring Withdrawal Symptoms—requires from one to three or more appointments, depending on the severity of the patient's withdrawal reaction. I met with all six patients—Claudia, Richard, Sarah, Gary, Daria, and Brent—within about a week of reducing their Paxil dose. I met with

Claudia and Richard only once to monitor their withdrawal symptoms after their initial dosage reductions, because they were having mild or no withdrawal symptoms. Brent and I met on day 5 and spoke by phone on day 7 when he went back up to 20 milligrams a day. We met again on day 8 to see how he was doing and on day 12, for a total of three appointments. Daria and I met on day 8. Her symptoms had already peaked the day before and were beginning to improve. So we only met once more, on day 13 at which point her symptoms were in the mild range. The number and frequency of meetings needs to be tailored to the patient's specific circumstances.

After all the patient's withdrawal symptoms have cleared, it is best to wait one to two weeks before moving on to Step 4, Making Additional Dosage Reductions, to give the patient time to fully recover from an episode of withdrawal. Since a typical withdrawal reaction lasts about two weeks, this means roughly one month between dosage reductions. If the patient's withdrawal reaction lasts longer than two weeks, then more than a month will elapse before the next dosage reduction. If the patient has no withdrawal symptoms, the month may be cut back to three weeks: It takes a week to establish that the patient is not having a withdrawal reaction and then one typically waits another two weeks.

Why wait one to two weeks? If the patient has had a moderate-to-severe withdrawal reaction, he will often be shaken up and exhausted by it and literally need two weeks to recover before attempting another reduction. But even when the patient has had a mild-to-moderate withdrawal reaction, waiting a week or two is a good idea. Even when patients only have mild-to-moderate symptoms or no symptoms at all, their brain cells are still readjusting to living with less of the drug. As discussed in Chapter 1, some antidepressant effects, like abnormal eye movements during sleep, can persist for over a year *after* the drug is stopped.[7] If some antidepressant effects can persist for more than a year after the drugs are stopped, giving the nervous system a month to adjust to each dosage reduction does not seem unreasonable.

In addition to physiologically "cushioning" brain cells by providing them with adequate time to readjust, waiting two weeks provides a psychological cushion as well. The two weeks allow patients to reestablish their physiological and their psychological equilibrium after an episode of antidepressant withdrawal. More than two weeks is not necessary unless the patient has had a particularly severe withdrawal reaction and wants longer to recover. But, these two extra weeks to recover are an important ingredient in successfully tapering patients off antidepressants. Making more frequent reductions produces a cumulative effect of rapidly lowering the antidepressant's level in the brain that can "catch up" with patients and increase their risk of more severe withdrawal reactions.

Of course, there are exceptions to every rule. If the patient has a good reason to want to get off an antidepressant quickly—like a severe, worrisome side effect—and has no withdrawal symptoms, then one might make the next reduction after just two weeks.

10

Step 4: Making Additional Dosage Reductions

Claudia, Richard, Sarah, Gary, Daria, and Brent are all now about a month into their antidepressant tapering programs. They have all recovered fully from whatever withdrawal symptoms they had after their initial dosage reductions. If we now examine each one's additional dosage reductions, we will see how a patient's reaction to each reduction becomes the basis on which one chooses the size of the next reduction.

As we have seen with these six patients' initial dosage reductions, the difficult part of tapering antidepressants is the unpredictability of people's withdrawal reactions and the tremendous variations one sees from one patient to the next. In an antidepressant tapering program, the goal is to establish a routine, or rhythm, of reasonable size dosage reductions at regular intervals, roughly once a month. Reasonable size dosage reductions are ones that produce mild withdrawal reactions or no withdrawal reactions at all.

For patients who have mild withdrawal reactions or no withdrawal reaction at all after the initial dosage reduction, the goal of establishing reasonable size dosage reductions has already been achieved. These patients can continue to follow the recommended dosage reductions in Table 6.2, "Recommended Tapering Programs for Today's Popular Antidepressants" (on page 93). This is true for the majority of patients tapering off antidepressants with the 5-Step Antidepressant Tapering Program, because the dosage reductions have been carefully chosen on the basis of experience with many patients.

Patients who have mild withdrawal reactions or no withdrawal reaction at all after the initial dosage reduction—like Claudia or Richard—simply make the next dosage reduction suggested in Table 6.2 (page 93). This is because once the pattern of a patient's withdrawal reaction to one of the dosage reductions in Table 6.2 is established, the pattern is likely to repeat itself after the next recommended reduction. That is, the patient is likely to have much the same symptoms with about the same level of severity. The timing of the symptoms—their onset, peak, and resolution—is also likely to repeat itself.

Patients who have moderate withdrawal reactions after the initial dosage reduction—like Sarah or Gary—need to proceed more slowly. They try a smaller reduction, one half the size of the next recommended dosage reduction in Table 6.2. For patients who continue to have moderate withdrawal reactions, one keeps making smaller and smaller dosage reductions, each time cutting the reduction in half again until one arrives at a dosage reduction that produces no withdrawal reaction or a mild withdrawal reaction and can therefore be repeated.

Patients who have a severe withdrawal reaction after the initial dosage reduction—like Daria and Brent—proceed even more slowly. They try a dosage reduction one-half to one-quarter the size of the next recommended dosage reduction in Table 6.2. For patients who continue to have severe withdrawal reactions, one keeps making smaller and smaller dosage reductions, each time cutting the reduction in half or to one-quarter until one arrives at a reduction that can be repeated because it produces a mild withdrawal reaction or no withdrawal reaction at all.

Moderate withdrawal reactions are somewhat of a gray zone. Some patients whose withdrawal reactions fall in the high end of the moderate range may want to follow the guidelines for severe withdrawal reactions and proceed more cautiously, or slowly. Conversely, some patients whose withdrawal reactions fall in the low end of the moderate range may want to follow the guidelines for mild withdrawal reactions and proceed more aggressively, or quickly.

The guidelines for making additional dosage reductions in the 5-Step Antidepressant Tapering Program are summarized in Table 10.1. Using these guidelines, one either:

- continues to make the dosage reductions outlined in Table 6.2, "Recommended Tapering Programs for Today's Popular Antidepressants"
- or, one customizes the size of reductions following the recommendations in Table 10.1.

**Table 10.1 GUIDELINES FOR MAKING ADDITIONAL
DOSAGE REDUCTIONS IN THE 5-STEP
ANTIDEPRESSANT TAPERING PROGRAM**

FOR PATIENTS WHO HAVE:	FOR THE NEXT REDUCTION:
No withdrawal reaction or a mild withdrawal reaction	Make the next recommended dosage reduction outlined in Table 6.2 (page 93).
A moderate withdrawal reaction	Make one-half of the next recommended dosage reduction outlined in Table 6.2. If moderate withdrawal reactions continue, keep cutting the reduction in half until arriving at a dosage reduction that can be repeated because it produces a mild withdrawal reaction or no withdrawal reaction at all.
A severe withdrawal reaction	Make one-half to one-quarter of the next recommended dosage reduction outlined in Table 6.2. If severe withdrawal reactions continue, keep cutting the reduction in half or to one-quarter the size until arriving at a dosage reduction that can be repeated because it produces a mild withdrawal reaction or no withdrawal reaction at all.

With these guidelines, the goal of establishing a routine of reasonable size dosage reductions at monthly intervals can usually be achieved by the second or third reduction, even for patients who have severe withdrawal reactions following the initial reduction.

As with any aspect of treatment, deciding on the size of dosage reductions is a collaboration between the doctor and the patient. Planning dosage reductions involves negotiating and agreeing to a reduction the patient is comfortable with, based on her reaction to the previous reduction. Indeed, in the end, the patient decides what size dosage reduction she is comfortable making. The doctor's role is to help the patient make a well-informed choice.

As discussed in Chapter 8, Making the Initial Dosage Reduction, some patients are exceptions to the rule and start their tapering programs with one-half the recommended initial dosage reduction. For example, patients with histories of severe antidepressant withdrawal reactions start with smaller initial reductions. When this is the case, if the patient has little or no withdrawal reaction after the initial dosage reduction, for the second dosage reduction, one may want to try a larger reduction to see if the patient can, in fact, follow the recommended tapering program.

As one continues on an antidepressant tapering program, one alternates between monitoring withdrawal symptoms after dosage reductions and making the next reduction. The same guidelines apply each time one monitors withdrawal symptoms and each time one plans the next dosage reduction. One continues in this fashion until one reaches the final reduction when the patient stops the drug altogether.

For each dosage reduction, both doctor and patient need to agree on the day when the patient is going to make the change. The doctor needs to be sure the patient has the right size pills and to give her a prescription if she does not. The patient also needs to be given a new set of daily checklists to last two to three weeks. With each new dosage reduction, the clock is reset to day 1. The patient also needs a new graph if she wishes to plot her reaction to this new dosage reduction. Finally, a specific follow-up appointment should be scheduled—day, date, and time—to evaluate and monitor the patient's withdrawal symptoms following this new reduction in the dose of the antidepressant.

To some extent, one is limited in how much one can fine tune dosage reductions by the pill sizes available for the particular antidepressant. With Paxil this means one can easily make 5- and 10-milligram reductions. More effort is required to make 2.5-milligram reductions that necessitate cutting 10-milligram pills into quarters. Cutting pills into smaller fragments becomes difficult and imprecise, so one only resorts to this when necessary. One has an even higher threshold for resorting to using the liquid forms of antidepressants, because they are so expensive and require carefully measuring doses in a dropper. One only uses the liquid form to achieve tiny dosage reductions for patients with severe withdrawal reactions who truly require it.

Some patients settle into a routine of comfortable dosage reductions once a month only to have it interrupted by a moderate to severe withdrawal reaction. The more severe reaction forces them to make smaller reductions, slowing down the pace of their tapers. Once again, these kinds of interruptions are unpredictable and part of the process of tapering antidepressants. One simply needs to be prepared for them and make adjustments if necessary.

Why might the routine of some patients be interrupted by a moderate to severe withdrawal reaction as they progress through the taper to lower and lower doses? If one is in a routine of repeating the same milligram size reduction, at lower and lower doses this constitutes a larger and larger percentage size reduction. A 10-milligram reduction from 40 to 30 milligrams a day is a 25 percent reduction. But another 10-milligram reduction from 30 to 20 milligrams a day is a 33 percent reduction. And the next 10-milligram reduction from 20 to 10 milligrams a day is a 50 percent reduction, twice the size of the original 25 percent reduction. For some patients, this requires an adjustment as they lower the dose.

The last dosage reduction, when the patient stops taking the antidepressant altogether, is unique, because the drug is now washing completely out of the patient's system. The next chapter is therefore devoted to the end-of-taper evaluation. By the time most patients reach the last dosage reduction, they are in a routine of reasonable size dosage reductions that produce mild withdrawal reactions or no withdrawal reaction at all. When this pattern has been established, for many patients, stopping the drug is unremarkable: The pattern repeats itself one final time. But for other patients, this is not the case: Stopping their antidepressant produces worse withdrawal symptoms than previous reductions, since the drug is now leaving their system completely. Earlier in the book, we discussed how brain cells adapt to antidepressants when patients first go on the drugs and how the cells readjust—how they dismantle their adaptations—when patients taper off. For some patients, stopping their antidepressant is a bigger adjustment than earlier dosage reductions. The bigger readjustment puts more strain on brain cells and therefore produces a more severe withdrawal reaction.

Obviously, a wide variety of dosage reductions and tapering schedules are possible depending on the particular antidepressant and dose one is taking at each stage in a tapering program. Many patients are able to taper off antidepressants relatively uneventfully with little or no withdrawal symptoms, while others have to endure painstakingly slow tapers because of severe withdrawal reactions.

With this overview of what is to come, let's look at the additional dosage reductions of the six patients whose antidepressant tapering programs we are following closely. Remember, Claudia, Richard, Sarah,

Gary, Daria, and Brent are all tapering off 20 milligrams a day of Paxil. After following these six patients through their entire tapering programs, you will be thoroughly familiar with how the 5-Step Antidepressant Tapering Program works, regardless of what antidepressant or dose you are on.

Claudia's Tapering Program After Having No Withdrawal Reaction

In psychotherapy and on Paxil, Claudia left an abusive relationship and rebuilt her life. After two years of treatment, when Claudia reduced her daily Paxil dose from 20 down to 10 milligrams, she had no withdrawal symptoms at all. Because she had no withdrawal reaction, after waiting a month Claudia made the next suggested dosage reduction in the recommended tapering program for Paxil: She reduced her daily dose from 10 to 0 milligrams; that is, she stopped the medication altogether.

Table 6.3 on page 96 summarizes the tapering programs of the six patients whose programs we are following closely. As seen in the table, because she had no withdrawal reaction after her initial dosage reduction, Claudia was able to follow the tapering program recommended for patients on 20 milligrams a day of Paxil, reducing her daily dose from 20 to 10 to 0 milligrams.

How did Claudia do off Paxil? Did stopping the drug go as smoothly as her initial dosage reduction? Claudia's end-of-taper evaluation is discussed in the next chapter, because it is a separate, distinct step in an antidepressant tapering program. Indeed, all six patients' end-of-taper evaluations are discussed in the next chapter.

Richard's Tapering Program After a Mild Withdrawal Reaction

Like Claudia, Richard was able to follow the recommended tapering program for patients on 20 milligrams a day of Paxil, as seen in Table 6.3. Richard is the documentary film director who became depressed when a fire destroyed the film he was editing for a prestigious film festival. After more than a year of treatment, Richard was no longer depressed and wanted to go off Paxil because it was making him sluggish and fatigued.

When Richard reduced his daily Paxil dose from 20 to 10 milligrams, he only had mild withdrawal symptoms: a tremor, blurred vision, and dizziness.

Since Richard had a mild withdrawal reaction, a month later he was able to make the next suggested dosage reduction for patients tapering off Paxil, from 10 down to 0 milligrams. This meant that, with his second dosage reduction, Richard stopped taking Paxil altogether.

Another patient in Richard's position might have elected to proceed more slowly. A patient who did not want to run the risk of a more severe tremor or more severe dizziness might have chosen a 5-milligram reduction instead. This is a judgment call ultimately up to the patient. Claudia's and Richard's tapering programs proceeded relatively uneventfully, as is the case for the majority patients following the guidelines of the 5-Step Antidepressant Tapering Program.

Sarah's Tapering Program After a Withdrawal Reaction in the Lower End of the Moderate Range

Sarah is the earth-mother in flowing scarves who lost her job because of alcoholism and developed panic attacks. After Sarah used Alcoholics Anonymous to become sober, I was able to put her on Paxil for the panic attacks. She also did a cognitive-behavioral therapy program to learn skills for managing her anxiety. Sarah wanted to go off Paxil because of severe sexual side effects.

Following her initial dosage reduction from 20 down to 10 milligrams a day, Sarah had psychiatric withdrawal symptoms—low energy, crying spells, insomnia, memory problems, and trouble concentrating—in the low end of the moderate range. Having had a moderate withdrawal reaction, Sarah was advised to slow her taper down by making a smaller dosage reduction than the one recommended in Table 6.2 (page 93). Since the next suggested dosage reduction is 10 milligrams, the next month Sarah made a dosage reduction half this size, to 5 milligrams reducing her daily dose from 10 down to 5 milligrams. With this smaller reduction, Sarah had a mild withdrawal reaction that lasted two weeks. After waiting an additional two weeks, Sarah made another 5-milligram reduction and stopped taking Paxil altogether. Sarah's tapering schedule is summarized in Table 6.3 (page 96): She reduced her daily Paxil dose from 20 to 10 to 5 to 0 milligrams, making the reductions about once a month.

Gary's Tapering Program After a Withdrawal Reaction in the Higher End of the Moderate Range

Gary is the young biotechnician dressed in all black who became depressed after his girlfriend broke up with him. After nine months of psychotherapy and Paxil, Gary was no longer depressed, in a new relationship, and wanted to go off the antidepressant because he was concerned about the long-term risks. When Gary reduced his daily Paxil dose from 20 to 10 milligrams, he had a withdrawal reaction in the high end of the moderate range. Gary experienced quite uncomfortable flu-like symptoms, dizziness, irritability, and "jumping" vision. Although he was able to endure this episode of antidepressant withdrawal, Gary did not want to repeat it. When we met to plan his next dosage reduction, we agreed he would reduce the dose more gradually by making a 5-milligram reduction, from 10 to 5 milligrams a day, following the guidelines for dosage reductions after moderate withdrawal reactions.

Since Gary had a withdrawal reaction in the high end of the moderate range, his case falls into somewhat of a gray zone. Another patient with a similar withdrawal reaction might have wanted to proceed even more conservatively by following the guidelines for dosage reductions after severe withdrawal reactions. This would have meant a 2.5-milligram reduction from 10 to 7.5 milligrams a day, instead of the 5-milligram reduction to 5 milligrams a day. This is a judgment call that is up to the individual patient.

Unlike Sarah, Gary's 5-milligram reduction produced another withdrawal reaction in the moderate range. So, Gary again adjusted the size of his next reduction, cutting the dosage reduction in half, to 2.5-milligrams. Gary finally had a mild withdrawal reaction after his 2.5-milligram reduction, so he repeated it for his next reduction and stopped taking Paxil altogether. Gary's tapering schedule is summarized in Table 6.3 (page 96): He reduced his daily Paxil dose from 20 to 10 to 5 to 2.5 to 0 milligrams, making the reductions about once a month. Gary made a total of four steps down in his Paxil dose before stopping the drug altogether, by comparison with Claudia's and Richard's two steps and Sarah's three.

Sarah and Gary both had moderate withdrawal reactions following their initial dosage reductions. Both made second dosage reductions that were one-half the size of the recommended dosage reduction. For Sarah, the smaller, 5-milligram reduction produced a mild withdrawal reaction so she could then repeat the 5-milligram size reduction. But for Gary, the 5-milligram reduction produced another moderate withdrawal reaction. So, for his next dosage reduction, Gary cut the reduction size in half again, to 2.5 milligrams. The 2.5-milligram reduction finally produced a mild withdrawal reaction, so he was able to repeat it, making another 2.5-milligram reduction. Gary's case illustrates an important point: If one continues to have moderate or severe withdrawal reactions, one continues to cut subsequent dosage reductions in half or in one-quarter until one arrives at a dosage reduction that can be repeated because it produces little or no withdrawal reaction.

Daria's Tapering Program After Her Severe Withdrawal Reaction

Daria is the Harvard College sophomore who developed psychosomatic concerns about her own health after her mother died of congestive heart failure. After being in treatment for ten months, Daria had made considerable progress grieving her mother and wanted to go off Paxil because she was gaining weight on the drug. After her initial dosage reduction, Daria had severe nausea, vomiting, abdominal pain, irritability, and depressed mood. Daria's withdrawal reaction was not quite severe enough to force her to go back up on the dose, but she still wanted to avoid such severe symptoms the next time.

To avoid a repeat of her severe withdrawal reaction, Daria made a smaller reduction the next time: a 2.5-milligram reduction from 10 to 7.5 milligrams a day. Following the guidelines for dosage reductions after severe withdrawal reactions, this was one-quarter the size of the recommended dosage reduction at this stage in tapering Paxil. With this considerably smaller reduction, Daria had a mild withdrawal reaction. Having found a comfortable size dosage reduction that caused a mild withdrawal reaction, going forward, Daria continued to make 2.5-milligram reductions.

Daria made her first two dosage reductions in July and August of the summer between her junior and senior years of college. She then put her tapering program on hold in September because she did not want to make a dosage reduction during her transition back to school. When the transition went well, in October and November Daria made two additional 2.5-milligram reductions. Each time she had withdrawal symptoms in the mild range. Once she was down to 2.5 milligrams a day, Daria did not go off the drug in December because of holidays and studying for exams. Instead, she waited until late January, after her exams were over.

Many patients tapering antidepressants will put their tapers on hold for a month or two while they get through a transition or a stressful period. I encourage patients to work their tapering programs around the rest of their lives. This is a sensible way to gradually go off the drugs. Daria made a total of five reductions before stopping the Paxil altogether. Daria's antidepressant tapering program is summarized in Table 6.3 (page 96): She made reductions in her daily dose from 20 to 10 to 7.5 to 5 to 2.5 to 0 milligrams.

Brent's Tapering Program After His Severe Withdrawal Reaction

Of the patients we have been following, Brent had the most difficult time weaning off Paxil. Brent is the young father who became depressed when he lost his job shortly after his son was born. Brent went through a grueling job search to land a new job. After settling in to it, Brent wanted to try going off Paxil because he was no longer depressed and had developed sexual side effects.

Brent had a severe withdrawal reaction following his initial reduction from 20 to 10 milligrams a day of Paxil. Indeed, Brent's dizziness and electric shock–like sensations were so severe that he was forced to go back up to 20 milligrams a day. Unnerved by such a severe reaction, Brent took several weeks to recover from it. After waiting two weeks after all his withdrawal symptoms had cleared, Brent was ready to try a smaller dosage reduction.

Following the guidelines for dosage reductions after severe withdrawal reactions, Brent's next dosage reduction was to be between 2.5 and 5 milligrams, one-quarter to one-half the recommended 10-milligram reduction. Brent objected to a 2.5-milligram reduction, saying that it was too small. Having "made no progress" with his first dosage reduction because he was forced to put his dose back up, Brent wanted to "press on" more aggressively. So, he tried a 5-milligram reduction, half the size of the recommended dosage reduction.

Unfortunately, Brent again had severe dizziness and imbalance although not as severe as the first time around. Despite being quite uncomfortable, this time Brent did not have to put his dose back up. Brent felt frustrated and demoralized when even a 5-milligram reduction produced a severe withdrawal reaction. However, I reassured him that we would just try a smaller, 2.5-milligram reduction as soon as he recovered from this episode of withdrawal.

For the next reduction, Brent tried lowering his daily dose from 15 down to 12.5 milligrams. With this small, 2.5-milligram reduction, Brent finally had a mild withdrawal reaction. From that point on, he was able to get into a routine, or rhythm, of making 2.5-milligram reductions every few weeks: 12.5 to 10 to 7.5 to 5 to 2.5 to 0. Each time, Brent would have about ten days of mild withdrawal symptoms and then we would wait ten days to two weeks for him to fully recover from the episode of withdrawal before making another reduction. Whenever possible, Brent made reductions every three weeks rather than once a month because he wanted to "make up for the lost time" of his first two dosage reductions. Once we found a dosage reduction that worked for him, as seen in Table 6.3 (page 96), Brent made a total of eight excruciatingly slow reductions in the dose before stopping Paxil altogether.

The Wide Variation in Antidepressant Tapering Programs

Looking at Table 6.3 and reflecting on Claudia's, Richard's, Sarah's, Gary's, Daria's, and Brent's antidepressant tapering programs, you can now appreciate how the flexibility of the 5-Step Antidepressant Tapering Program works. The recommended schedule for tapering off 20 milligrams a day of Paxil is to reduce the dose from 20 to 10 to 0 milligrams, making reductions about once a month. Claudia and Richard both had mild withdrawal reactions or no withdrawal reaction at all and were able to follow the recommended program. Their experience is typical of the majority of patients following the 5-Step Antidepressant Tapering Program, because the recommended dosage reductions are chosen to be reasonable in size based on experience with many patients.

Sarah and Gary had moderate withdrawal reactions and had to slow their tapers down. Gary had to slow his taper down more than Sarah, because he had another moderate withdrawal reaction after his second dosage reduction even though it was only 5 milligrams in size. Sarah and Gary slowed their tapers down using the guidelines for customizing dosage reductions, tailoring them to the individual patient.

Daria and Brent had to slow their tapers down even more because of severe withdrawal reactions. Daria's initial withdrawal reaction was not quite severe enough to force her to go back up on the dose. So, she "made it" from 20 to 10 milligrams a day with her initial dosage reduction. Thereafter, she reduced her dose painstakingly slowly by 2.5 milligrams at a time. Brent made "no progress" with his initial dosage reduction because he was forced back up to 20 milligrams a day. He tried a 5-milligram reduction to 15 milligrams a day but again had a severe withdrawal reaction, although not severe enough to force him to go back up on the dose. Thereafter, Brent reduced his dose very gradually by 2.5 milligrams at a time.

As these six patients illustrate, tapering off antidepressants is a trial-and-error process. If one has mild withdrawal reactions or no withdrawal reactions at all, one can simply follow the recommended tapering schedule for your antidepressant. If, on the other hand, you have moderate to severe withdrawal reactions, then you customize your dosage reductions making smaller and smaller reductions until you arrive at one that can be repeated because it produces a mild withdrawal reaction or no withdrawal reaction at all. In the 5-Step Antidepressant Tapering Program, the recommended tapering schedules work for the majority of patients while, at the same time, the program's flexibility can accommodate even the most difficult cases. The same principles and guidelines used by these six patients to taper off 20 milligrams a day of Paxil can be applied to tapering off any dose of any of today's popular antidepressants.

11

Step 5: The End-of-Taper Evaluation

Claudia, Richard, Sarah, Gary, Daria, and Brent all met with me for end-of-taper evaluations after their final dosage reductions when they stopped Paxil altogether. All patients need to be monitored for withdrawal reactions after their final dosage reduction. By the time most patients stop their antidepressant, they are in a routine of reasonable sized dosage reductions that produce no withdrawal symptoms or mild withdrawal reactions. For these patients, stopping the drug is uneventful. But other patients have worse withdrawal symptoms, because the drug is now washing completely out of their systems. An antidepressant tapering program is not over until the patient stops the drug and either:

• proves to have no withdrawal reaction, or
• recovers fully from whatever withdrawal symptoms occur

As with earlier dosage reductions, end-of-taper evaluations are scheduled to coincide with when withdrawal symptoms are most likely to appear. For patients stopping Paxil or one of the other shorter-acting antidepressants, the ideal time to schedule a follow-up evaluation is about three to seven days after stopping the drug. For patients stopping the long-acting antidepressant Prozac, the best time is two to three weeks. If, at that time, the patient is having a withdrawal reaction, another evaluation should be scheduled within days to a week, depending on the severity of the symptoms. However, even if the patient is having no withdrawal symptoms, a second meeting is scheduled. For patients stopping Paxil or another of the shorter-acting antidepressants, this second meeting is scheduled for two to three weeks after the patient stopped the drug. For patients stopping Prozac, this second meeting is scheduled for five to six weeks after the patient has stopped the drug. At that point, either the patient has had:

- No withdrawal symptoms
- Mild-to-moderate withdrawal symptoms that may have already cleared
- A severe withdrawal reaction that has forced the patient to resume taking the antidepressant

Four of the six patients whose antidepressant tapering programs we have been following closely—Claudia, Sarah, Brent, and Daria—made their final dosage reduction and stopped Paxil uneventfully. Claudia had no withdrawal reaction, the same as after her previous dosage reduction. Sarah, Brent, and Daria had mild withdrawal reactions, as they had after their previous reductions.

In Brent's case, because he had a history of severe withdrawal reactions earlier in his taper, I used a technique I have used with other patients to cushion his final dosage reduction. Since Brent was going to be taking 2.5 milligrams a day of Paxil for the final month before he stopped the drug, he precut all thirty of the 2.5 milligram pieces he was going to need. To do so, he cut 10-milligram pills into quarters. Of course the pieces varied in size: The largest fragments probably approached 3 milligrams in size, while the smallest fragments were closer to 2 milligrams. Brent lined the pieces up from largest to smallest. Taking them in this order, from large to small, served to make reducing his dose even more gradual. The array of smaller and smaller pill fragments also formed a graphic, visual representation of the end of Brent's taper. Taking the pill fragments from large to small cushioned Brent's final dosage reduction and contributed to his having a mild withdrawal reaction.

Two of the six patients—Richard and Gary—had more severe withdrawal reactions when they stopped Paxil than they had had after their previous reductions. After his initial dosage reduction from 20 to 10 milligrams a day, Richard had a mild withdrawal reaction with a tremor, blurred vision, and dizziness. Since he tolerated the mild withdrawal reaction comfortably, Richard followed the recommended tapering program and stopped the drug altogether.

I met Richard for his end-of-taper evaluation four days after he stopped taking Paxil. To his surprise, Richard was having a worse withdrawal reaction after stopping the drug. This time the dizziness, blurred vision, and "cotton wool" feeling in his head affected Richard's ability to function. However, his symptoms did not become incapacitating or severe. Richard did not have to go back on the Paxil. His withdrawal reaction gradually improved over the course of two weeks.

During his antidepressant tapering program, Gary had two moderate withdrawal reactions that forced him to slow his taper down to a 2.5-milligram reduction that had produced a mild withdrawal reaction. When he made a final 2.5-milligram reduction and stopped taking Paxil, Gary unexpectedly had a worse withdrawal reaction than he had after his previous reduction of the same size.

When I met with him five days after he stopped the antidepressant, Gary was having a moderate withdrawal reaction that included dizziness, flu-like aches and pains, and irritability. When I met with him again the following week, Gary's withdrawal symptoms had peaked and were subsiding. His withdrawal reaction did not become severe enough to force him to go back on the medication.

Examples like Richard's and Gary's make the case for why it is so important to evaluate patients after they stop taking their antidepressant, in the same way they are evaluated after each of their earlier dosage reductions. Richard's and Gary's withdrawal reactions after stopping Paxil were worse than their reactions after the previous reduction of the same size. If Richard's or Gary's withdrawal reaction had become severe, it would have forced them to go back on the drug. A patient in Richard's or Gary's position should not be on his own, without medical supervision, trying to monitor his own symptoms and unsure what to do.

Patients Who Have to Temporarily Go Back on Their Antidepressant

Most patients who follow the 5-Step Antidepressant Tapering Program have no withdrawal reaction at all when they stop the drug completely or have mild to moderate withdrawal reactions that they tolerate relatively comfortably. Patients who taper carefully off their antidepressants usually do not have severe withdrawal reactions that force them to go back on the antidepressant. They may have a worse reaction than they had to the previous reductions of the same size, like Richard and Gary, but not severe enough to force them back on the drug.

When one sees patients temporarily forced to go back on their antidepressant, it is typically because they either stopped the drug abruptly or they tapered off it too quickly. Two new patients who we have not previously discussed illustrate this point. As seen in Table 11.1, Paul stopped 20 milligrams a day of Paxil "cold turkey" and had a severe withdrawal reaction that forced him to go back on the antidepressant. After he recovered from the "shock" of a withdrawal reaction so severe that he had to restart the drug, Paul tapered off Paxil more slowly. He made 5-milligram reductions at a time, each of which produced mild, tolerable withdrawal reactions.

Cases like Paul's are an important reminder that patients should not abruptly stop antidepressants at doses equivalent to 20 milligrams a day of Paxil or higher. Earlier in the book, John—the Harvard undergraduate who got in trouble with the law and could have been expelled from college—had also stopped just 20 milligrams a day of Paxil. When one looks at cases like Claudia's and Richard's—patients who have mild withdrawal reactions or no withdrawal reaction at all tapering their daily Paxil doses from 20 to 10 to 0 milligrams—one might be tempted to try stopping

Table 11.1 TAPERING PROGRAMS FOR TWO PATIENTS WHO HAD TO RESTART THEIR ANTIDEPRESSANTS AND TAPERED OFF MORE SLOWLY

RECOMMENDED	PAUL	LOUISE
20	20	40
10	0	20
0	*20*	10
	15	5
	10	0
	5	*5*
	0	2.5
		0

The step at which the patient had to restart the antidepressant is indicated by asterisks and bold type

20 milligrams a day without tapering off. But one runs the risk of a severe withdrawal reaction, like Paul's or, worse, like John's. Even pharmaceutical companies like GlaxoSmithKline now recommend tapering the drugs.

Louise tapered off 40 milligrams a day of Paxil, as seen in Table 11.1. Louise made dosage reductions relatively frequently, every two-and-a-half to three weeks, rather than once a month, because she was anxious to get her taper "over with." Despite having a moderate withdrawal reaction after the initial reduction in her daily dose, from 40 down to 20 milligrams, Louise insisted on pushing ahead with the next recommended dosage reduction from 20 to 10 milligrams. When Louise had another moderate withdrawal reaction, she finally slowed her taper, making a 5-milligram reduction in her daily dose from 10 to 5 milligrams. Still, when she had yet another moderate withdrawal reaction, she declined to make a 2.5-milligram reduction, because this would have meant quartering 10-milligram pills into 2.5-milligram pieces. Louise did not want the "hassle" of quartering pills and was confident she could "survive" one last moderate withdrawal reaction.

The pace of Louise's tapering program caught up with her when she went off Paxil: Louise had a severe withdrawal reaction that forced her to go back on the drug. After she recovered from the episode of severe withdrawal, Louise resumed her taper at a slower pace, making 2.5-milligram reductions once a month. Louise's case illustrates an important point: Accelerating the pace of a tapering program—by making dosage reductions too frequently and/or by making dosage reductions that are too large—can backfire, causing the patient to have a severe, incapacitating withdrawal reaction.

A severe withdrawal reaction at the end of an antidepressant tapering program does *not* indicate that the patient needs to stay on the drug. As with earlier dosage reductions, the symptoms are drug-induced withdrawal phenomena, not a depressive relapse. After temporarily going back on the medication, the patient simply needs to extend the taper and wean off the drug more slowly. When patients have to go back on antidepressants, they reinstate the previous dose, as Paul and Louise did.

Longer-Term Follow-up After Stopping an Antidepressant

If at all possible, patients should be followed at least once a month for a number of months after completing an antidepressant tapering program to be sure they are fine off the medication. Some patients who have recently stopped antidepressants are acutely sensitive to the ups and downs of their days. They need to be monitored to see how they are doing and to provide support and reassurance. If they have a bad day, they need to ask themselves: Did I have bad days while I was on the antidepressant? Most patients will answer yes to the question. When monitoring patients for relapse, a return of their original psychiatric condition, one is looking for real evidence of deterioration over longer periods of time—weeks rather than days. In my experience, few people relapse and have to go back on antidepressants if, after careful consideration, they and their doctors felt they no longer need the medication and if they tapered slowly off their drug following the guidelines of the 5-Step Antidepressant Tapering Program.

When patients are in ongoing psychotherapy with their psychiatrist after stopping their antidepressant, monitoring how well they are doing is relatively easy, since the psychiatrist is seeing them regularly and talking about their emotional lives in some depth. If the patient is not in psychotherapy with the psychiatrist who prescribed the drug, then the therapist, usually a psychologist or social worker, may be the clinician seeing the patient most frequently and monitoring her mental health the most closely. Ideally, the patient would still check in with the doctor once a month for several months. Some patients are not in any other form of treatment and decline ongoing follow-up once the tapering program is over. These patients are encouraged to return at any time in the future if they have questions or concerns.

Claudia, Richard, Sarah, Gary, Daria, and Brent all continued to see me for longer-term follow-up after their antidepressant tapering programs were complete. None of them has needed to go back on Paxil despite challenges and crises in their lives.

Claudia

Claudia was able to follow the recommended program for patients tapering off 20 milligrams a day of Paxil. Since she had no withdrawal reactions, Claudia completed her tapering program in less than two months. If Claudia had started from a Paxil dose higher than 20 milligrams a day or if she had tried to go off the 20-milligram dose cold turkey, she might well have had withdrawal reactions. In any case, she felt fortunate to have such a relatively easy time going off the drug.

Like many women who have been in abusive relationships, Claudia did not enter into a new relationship for a number of years. She found that dating men was difficult in the early years while she was trying to put her life back together. She is finally in a new relationship, but is still working through her "trust issues" with men.

Richard

Richard, too, was able to follow the recommended tapering program and completed the program in less than two months. Off Paxil, Richard's "sluggishness" and fatigue cleared up. Richard hoped to be reinvited to the film festival the following year but was not. Still, he did not become depressed. Indeed, he was pleased to be off the Paxil to "prove" to himself that he could weather the disappointment without the drug. He continues to make films and to teach documentary filmmaking in Boston.

Sarah

Sarah had moderate withdrawal reactions and took a total of three months to complete her antidepressant tapering program. Off Paxil, her severe sexual dysfunction cleared. For Sarah, AA became the focus of her ongoing treatment, or recovery. With the skills she learned in the cognitive-behavioral program, she was able to manage periodic bouts of anxiety. Sarah has strong administrative skills and quickly found a new job once she was back on her feet. She checked in with me monthly for a number of months, once she finished her antidepressant tapering program.

A year after I stopped seeing Sarah, she came back to see me when she relapsed and began drinking again after her father died. Once again, she relied more on AA than on me to reestablish her sobriety. She has been doing well for three years now.

Gary

While Gary had not had any side effects while on Paxil, he had not wanted to stay on the drug indefinitely if he no longer needed it. Gary's experience of withdrawal reactions in the high end of the moderate range convinced him he had "made the right decision" to go off the Paxil. "Paxil obviously had a powerful effect on my brain," says Gary, "since it caused me to have such serious withdrawal reactions."

Gary stayed in psychotherapy with me for an additional six months. He gradually tapered off the therapy, shifting to every other week and then to once a month. He and the girlfriend he was seeing at the time have since broken up, Gary told me when I contacted him to get his permission to include him in this book. After dating a number of women for briefer periods of time, he is now in the "most serious" relationship of his life. Indeed, he expects to soon become engaged.

Daria

Daria took seven months to taper off Paxil because she put her tapering program "on hold" more than once due to her busy schedule with school and exams. Daria wanted to go off Paxil because she was steadily gaining weight on the antidepressant. Once Daria was down to 5 milligrams a day of Paxil, she stopped gaining weight and her weight stabilized. After she stopped the Paxil altogether, she gradually lost the weight through dieting and exercising.

Daria continued to see me for much of her remaining year of college. The loss of her mother had been traumatic and, with her family in Chicago, she was appreciative of the support. Daria majored in economics and is now thriving in a demanding graduate school program.

Brent

In total, tapering off Paxil took Brent six and a half frustrating months. Once he was off Paxil, Brent's sexual side effects cleared. After his antidepressant tapering program was finished, Brent continued in psychotherapy with me for a number of months. He wanted to consolidate the insights he had gained in psychotherapy. Brent's own father had been an alcoholic who abandoned his family, so when Brent lost his job, he was "paralyzed" by the prospect of not being able to support his young family. Although he was pleased his new job was working out well, the experience had brought back many memories of growing up in an alcoholic family. Working through the memories allowed Brent to convince himself that although he was temporarily unemployed, he was not an alcoholic parent unable to meet his family's needs.

Brent has been off Paxil for several years. He has not had any return of his depression, despite several crises around his son's health and the acquisition of his company by a much larger one.

The Wide Variations in the Duration of Antidepressant Tapering Programs

As we conclude following the antidepressant tapering programs of Claudia, Richard, Sarah, Gary, Daria, and Brent, notice once again in Table 6.3 on page 96 and in Figure 9.1 on pages 145–146 how they illustrate the wide variation seen from one patient to the next. Patients like Claudia and Richard, who start their taper at 20 milligrams a day of Paxil and who have mild withdrawal reactions or no withdrawal reaction at all, can complete their tapering programs in less than two months. Patients who start their tapers at high doses or patients who have moderate withdrawal reactions, like Gary and Sarah, typically take two to four months to taper off their antidepressants. And patients like Brent and Daria, who have severe withdrawal reactions that force them to taper their antidepressants extremely slowly, take longer than four months to wean off the drugs. These six patients were chosen to illustrate the wide range of withdrawal reactions and tapering programs seen in different patients tapering off the same dose of an antidepressant. At the same time, they represent fairly typical cases and do not include patients like Karen in Chapter 4, who had to be hospitalized because she developed life-threatening Celexa withdrawal symptoms, including auditory hallucinations telling her to kill herself and her family; or Helen in the BBC exposés, who weaned herself off Paxil painstakingly slowly, using a dropper to measure out tiny dosage reductions of the liquid form of the drug; or Andy in the next chapter, who had severe Effexor withdrawal reactions and had to make tiny dosage reductions of just a milligram at a time.

Variations on the Theme: Tapering Off Other Antidepressants

Regardless of the antidepressant and dose you are taking at the start of a tapering program, the same guidelines and principles apply. Unless you fall into one of the exceptions to the rule discussed in Chapter 8, working with your doctor, simply find the dose of your antidepressant in Table 6.2 on page 93 and make the suggested initial dosage reduction. As long as you have mild withdrawal reactions, or no withdrawal reaction at all, continue to make the series of recommended dosage reductions in Table

6.2. If you have moderate or severe withdrawal reactions, slow your taper down by customizing the dosage reductions according to the guidelines in Table 10.1 on page 157. Regardless of which one of today's popular antidepressants you are on, the same principles apply. If you are taking an older antidepressant (a tricyclic or a monoamine oxidase inhibitor) see the relevant Appendix at the back of the book.

12

Tapering Children Off Antidepressants

"I can only make one-milligram reductions at a time in my Effexor dose," sixteen-year-old Andy reported. When I first met him, Andy had been tapering off Effexor painstakingly slowly for months. I found Andy an extremely personable, articulate teenager whose life had been taken over by Effexor withdrawal. Andy is tall and athletic-looking with thick wavy black hair. He has a ready smile and wry sense of humor, which helped him through the ordeal. He and his family live in Arlington, Massachusetts, right next to Cambridge. He has two younger sisters.

"You can only make reductions of one milligram at a time?" I inquired.

"Even with such small reductions, I'm nauseous much of the time. But if I make reductions any larger, even a couple of milligrams, I have terrible nausea, vomiting, headaches, and dizziness."

"How do you make such small dosage reductions? Effexor pills are capsules with hundreds of tiny beads. Effexor doesn't come in a liquid form to facilitate such small dosage reductions. How do you make one-milligram reductions with 75-milligram capsules?"

"I count out the beads."

"You count the beads?"

"There are 180 beads in a 75-milligram capsule of Effexor. I started tapering this way from 112.5 milligrams, a 75-milligram capsule plus a

37.5-milligram capsule a day. So, I started at 270 beads a day. I reduce the number by two beads at a time to make dosage reductions."

"How excruciating."

"It's the only way I can do it. I'm down to 140 beads a day."

"How long have you been doing this?"

"Four months. And I'm not even half way through."

Said Andy's mother, Beth, the first time I met her: "We've been everywhere trying to get help with Effexor withdrawal and haven't been able to find it. We've been to our pediatrician and to child psychiatrists. Doctors don't seem to know what to do. We even went to one of the best-known specialists in child psychopharmacology at the Massachusetts General Hospital and he said Andy wasn't depressed and didn't need the Effexor, but that he didn't know how to help get Andy off it."

Despite the slow taper, during the four months Andy had been in virtually continuous Effexor withdrawal with waxing and waning nausea, vomiting, and diarrhea. A sophomore in high school, Andy had missed days, even whole weeks, of school because of the withdrawal symptoms. His grades had suffered. A good athlete, he had been forced to give up sports. Even working out at the gym had become impossible: The nausea was worsened by the movement involved in lifting weights or aerobic exercise.

"How often do you make dosage reductions?" I asked Andy.

"Every one to three days, depending on how nauseous I'm feeling. Effexor withdrawal is ruining my sophomore year in high school. I've got to get off the drug by this summer. I have to be off it for my junior year so I'm back to normal for school, taking SATs, applying to college, and everything."

Andy reported that he had to take his Effexor dose "like clockwork" at the same time each day, in the early evening, or else he went into severe withdrawal: "If I'm an hour late, I start to get terrible nausea, vomiting, and diarrhea. Effexor withdrawal is like having someone hold a gun to your head and say: 'Take this drug, or else!' "

Said his mother: "Andy's life and our whole family life revolves around managing his withdrawal from Effexor. It's been a nightmare."

Effexor has the shortest half-life of today's antidepressants, just five hours.[1] Young children are even more vulnerable to antidepressant withdrawal than adults because they are faster metabolizers of the drugs.[2] As a result, antidepressants are inactivated and wash out of the body even more quickly in children than adults.

Andy first went on Effexor during the summer between his freshman and sophomore years. He had been distressed and in therapy for several months after a difficult breakup with his girlfriend. He was also in the midst of moving from one school to another, a difficult transition for anyone in high school.

After a month on 75 milligrams a day of Effexor, Andy wanted to go off the drug. The Effexor was not helping and it was causing severe side effects. On the drug, Andy was sweating profusely, a recognized side effect of antidepressants. Andy felt "numb," "distant," and "detached" emotionally, which many patients report on antidepressants.[3] Andy also felt so fatigued on Effexor that he was "dragging" himself through the day. This became a serious problem in September when he returned to school. Andy wanted to go off Effexor, but his psychiatrist convinced him to stay on the drug and, indeed, to try a higher dose to see if it worked. The psychiatrist switched Andy's dose to the evening so the fatigue would coincide with when he was sleeping, and increased his dose to 150 milligrams a day.

Andy had a bad reaction to the higher dose. He became tense, irritable, hostile, and aggressive, all recognized side effects of antidepressants, especially in the early weeks after the drugs are started or the dose is increased or decreased.[4] This cluster of antidepressant side effects together with becoming suicidal is why the FDA has issued warnings and why the British MHRA has virtually banned many antidepressants for children under the age of eighteen, as discussed earlier in the book.[5]

Andy did not become suicidal on 150 milligrams a day of Effexor, but he did become extremely hostile and irritable. His irritability reached a peak one night when he was backing the car out of the garage and hit the frame of the garage door, bumping the fender. "He came into the house in a rage," says his father, Lewis. "He was enraged with himself, the car, the garage door. . . . We couldn't calm him down." Says his mother: "This wasn't the kid we'd known for sixteen years. He was a different person on the higher dose of Effexor."

Andy's parents became really concerned when he began punching holes in walls. When they approached him to try to restrain him, Andy fled the house and was missing for over an hour. His father drove around frantically looking for him while his mother waited at home in case he returned. Finally, Andy called, apologetic and distraught. "I picked him up and drove around with him for ages calming him down," says Beth. Says Andy of the incident: "After that, I was determined to get off the

Effexor. I had a complete personality change on the higher dose of the drug."

Andy's psychiatrist explained that he would have to taper off the Effexor and suggested reducing his daily dose from 150 down to 75 milligrams. When he reduced his dose, Andy had severe nausea, vomiting, headaches, dizziness, chills, insomnia, fatigue, and difficulty concentrating. He was bedridden for days, missed a full week of school, and was ultimately forced to go back up on the dose to 112.5 milligrams a day.

For Andy's next dosage reduction, he tried removing five beads from an Effexor capsule, a reduction of about 2 milligrams. Even this was too large a reduction and made Andy quite ill. To combat the withdrawal symptoms, he tried a host of over-the-counter drugs, none of which worked, including Benadryl, Dramamine, Pepto-Bismol, and Tums. He even tried the prescription antacid Zantac to no avail. "I was really sick for most of the late fall while we were still reducing the dose by five beads, or about two milligrams, at a time," says Andy. "One weekend I went to New York to visit friends. The trip had been planned for months and I insisted on going because I had been looking forward to it so much. But in the middle of the weekend, I had to come home, I was so sick." Says his mother: "When he came back from New York, Andy looked so drained, pale, and discouraged. He was so nauseous he could barely hold down enough liquid to take the Effexor pill, but we were terrified that if he didn't take the Effexor he'd feel so much worse."

Andy's family was scheduled to go on a vacation over the Christmas break. "I was afraid I wouldn't be able to fly in a plane because of the nausea," says Andy. "That's when we discovered wristbands for motion sickness. They were the first thing that helped." The wristbands apply pressure to points on the palm side of the wrist and help reduce the nausea and dizziness of motion sickness. By wearing the wristbands and making even smaller, 1-milligram reductions at a time, by January most of the vomiting and diarrhea were gone. Andy still had significant nausea virtually all the time. And, mysteriously, on some days the nausea was worse and the vomiting and diarrhea returned. This was a mystery because Andy was making the same size dosage reductions consistently. Why would the same reduction be causing worse withdrawal symptoms on some days and not others?

Throughout this time, Andy was missing days of school. He told his guidance counselor and teachers what was going on so they would understand his absences. Hanging out with friends after school was difficult because he always had to rush home to take his Effexor at the same exact time, with food. Because Andy was nauseous so much of the time, the only food that appealed to him were high carbohydrate foods, so he had gained a considerable amount of weight. In the midwinter, Andy also began acupuncture treatments for the nausea, which helped. The acupuncturist placed needles in his wrists, abdomen, and forehead. After six weeks of acupuncture, he began taking homeopathic treatments prescribed by the acupuncturist. Some patients seek out these kinds of alternative treatments for antidepressant withdrawal symptoms. When patients find the treatments helpful, I am generally supportive of them as an adjunct to the 5-Step Antidepressant Tapering Program.

By the time I met Andy, he was already on the regimen of tiny, one-milligram dosage reductions every one to three days, depending on how nauseous he felt. He was wearing the motion sickness wristbands, getting acupuncture, and starting the homeopathic treatments. I suggested that adding a low dose of Prozac might blunt the severe Effexor withdrawal, but Andy was reluctant to add another antidepressant given his terrible experience with Effexor.

In late winter, Andy solved the mystery of why the apparently same sized dosage reductions were producing varying degrees of withdrawal symptoms.

"Not all Effexor capsules have the same number of beads," Andy reported. "I've been counting the beads I removed, not realizing that left a variable number of beads."

"So, while overall your dose has been going down over months, on a day-to-day basis it's been going up and down?"

"That's what I realized."

"Which explains your roller coaster symptoms."

"Now I'm counting the number of beads that I actually take. It's even more of a pain, but that way I know for sure my dose is decreasing."

As we worked together, Andy noticed that the nausea was worse in the morning, when he got out of bed and began moving around at the beginning of the day. With a letter from me to his school, he negotiated coming in later and making up an art class at the end of the day. He also found new motion sickness wristbands that delivered electrical impulses to pressure points on his wrists and were even more effective.

With the tiny dosage reductions, motion sickness wristbands, acupuncture, homeopathic treatments, and change in schedule Andy was feeling a little better and thought he might be able to play baseball, his favorite sport, in the spring. He made the junior varsity team and had high hopes that playing on the team would bring him a sense of normality. Unfortunately, Andy's hopes were soon dashed. When he had to miss practices because of the nausea, his coach was not sympathetic. When practices or games ran late, Andy could not get home fast enough to take his Effexor dose on time and would start to get sicker.

One day, when his baseball game was rescheduled to the early evening, Andy ran home to take his Effexor before the game, fearing that if he waited until after the game it would be too late and he would become too sick to play. Said Andy's mother: "What a way to live, always having to worry about when you're going to take a pill." Added Andy: "I feel like an addict whose life revolves around his drug."

Despite his best efforts, Andy was not able to complete the baseball season. After missing a number of practices and games, he was forced to quit the team. The loss had ramifications far beyond the one season. "That's the end of my baseball career," Andy lamented. "I have to give up hope of making the varsity team next year. I'll fall behind everyone else after missing this year, so there's no way I'll make varsity in high school." This was a serious blow.

Getting down to the 37.5 milligram Effexor capsule in the spring felt like a milestone for Andy. He also added vitamin C and a B complex vitamin to his regimen, which he felt helped. In June, Andy had to slow his taper down even more to feel well enough to study for his exams at the end of the school year. Over the summer, he finally managed to stop the drug altogether. The weekend after Andy stopped the Paxil he became suicidal and violent, punching holes in the walls of his home. "That was the low point of the taper," says Andy. "That's when I hit bottom. At the time I never would have believed how much better I'd feel after I'd been off the drug just a few weeks. It's important for people going through severe withdrawal reactions to know that, so when they hit bottom they know other people have gotten through it."

Andy was only on Effexor three months when he first tried to reduce his dose. His slow taper off Effexor took three times as long: nine months. "I wish the doctor knew to warn me," Andy shook his head. Not all children experience withdrawal as severe as Andy's. Like adults, children vary in how vulnerable they are to antidepressant withdrawal reactions, but on the whole, they are more vulnerable than adults. While Andy is the first patient I have treated who had to make such tiny dosage reductions, I regularly receive inquiries from patients, parents, and doctors across the country trying to cope with similar, severe withdrawal re-actions. Andy's case is like Helen's in "The Secrets of Paxil," the British Broadcasting Corporation's exposé on Paxil withdrawal.[6] Helen is a twenty-two-year-old graduate student in London who weaned herself off Paxil painstakingly slowly, making tiny dosage reductions with a dropper and the liquid form of the drug.

Says Andy's mother of their ordeal: "My advice to parents with chil-dren on antidepressants is: Beware, tapering the drug may take a long time. It's wrenching to watch children go through months of uncomfort-able withdrawal. But they need you to be strong, resourceful, and sup-portive to help them get through it."

If you are a parent who picked up the book and went straight to this chapter, be sure to read the rest of the book. As described in the chapters detailing the 5-Step Antidepressant Tapering Program, patients vary widely in how mild or severe their withdrawal reactions are. Some pa-tients experience little or no withdrawal symptoms while others experi-ence severe withdrawal reactions like Andy's.

Since children are more vulnerable than adults to antidepressant withdrawal reactions, several modifications to the 5-Step Antidepressant Tapering Program should be made in the early stages of a child's taper:

- Start with smaller initial dosage reductions—my recommendation is 50 percent
- Be prepared to be extremely flexible on the size and timing of dosage reductions
- Monitor children even more closely

When tapering children under the age of eighteen off antidepressants, the initial dosage reduction should be one-half the recommended initial dosage reductions in Table 6.2 (page 93). If, despite the small reduction, a child still has moderate to severe withdrawal reactions, then, using the guidelines of the 5-Step Antidepressant Tapering Program, keep trying smaller and smaller dosage reductions until you find a comfortable size reduction that can be repeated. In Andy's case, he made extraordinarily small dosage reductions of just one milligram at relatively short intervals, every one to three days. He could not tolerate larger dosage reductions, and if he waited a longer time between reductions, it could have literally taken him years to get off the drug.

If after an initial, small dosage reduction a child has no withdrawal reaction, then the next time you may want to try one of the larger, recommended dosage reductions in Table 6.2 (page 93). Customizing the dosage reductions for children requires discussion and close collaboration between the patient, parents, and doctor.

Children should be monitored even more closely than adults, especially in the early stages of an antidepressant tapering program. They should be seen as close to weekly as possible, at least until they establish a routine of reasonable size dosage reductions at regular intervals. Parents need to be well educated about all the possible symptoms of antidepressant withdrawal so they can monitor their children closely at home. When necessary, parents should be in regular telephone contact with the doctor between meetings. In my experience treating adolescents, they can become even more discouraged than adults by severe withdrawal reactions and painstakingly slow tapers. Children tapering antidepressants need all the support and encouragement they can get from the doctor. Taking nine months, the better part of a year, to taper off an antidepressant seems like an eternity to children who have less experience than adults with persevering in the pursuit of long-range goals.

If you are a parent reading this book, be prepared to be resourceful and inventive, as Andy's mother was, as you support your child through antidepressant withdrawal. If necessary, make a few of your own appointments with the doctor for support and encouragement in surviving the ordeal.

The larger question of whether antidepressants should be prescribed to children continues to be controversial. The British MHRA has all but banned many antidepressants for children under the age of eighteen because pharmaceutical company studies found the drugs did not work in children and caused a range of dangerous, overstimulating side effects, including agitation, sleeplessness, hostility, aggression, and suicidality.[7] The British based their conclusions on all of the pharmaceutical company data, both published and unpublished. Prescribing antidepressants to children is controversial in part because the published studies based on carefully selected data do not tell the full story.[8] Even published studies have been found to misrepresent the data on which they are based, exaggerating the benefits and minimizing the risks of the drugs.[9]

As I finish writing this book, the controversy over prescribing antidepressants to children under the age of eighteen continues to be debated in this country. In October 2004, the FDA upgraded its warning on antidepressants making children suicidal to the highest level possible: a prominent black box warning.[10] Still, a January 2004 study by Thomas Moore at the George Washington University Medical Center found that "89 percent of children" taking an antidepressant drug were taking it "for a medical use for which there was no evidence that it was FDA-approved."[11] Moore's study was based on the Center for Disease Control's National Ambulatory Medical Care Survey and National Hospital Ambulatory Medical Care Survey.[12] These two major government surveys tracked patterns of antidepressant drug use from 1998 through 2001.

Patients being given prescription drugs for conditions for which the drugs are not approved by the FDA is called "off-label" prescribing. Only Prozac is approved for depressed children by the FDA.[13] Only Prozac, Zoloft, and Luvox are approved for children with obsessive-compulsive disorder (OCD).[14] Prescriptions for Prozac for conditions other than depression and OCD, prescriptions for Zoloft and Luvox for conditions other than OCD, and prescriptions for the other antidepressants for children for any condition are all off-label. Like adults, children are prescribed antidepressants for a host of conditions from school phobia to attention deficit disorder to headaches. The antidepressant most commonly prescribed to children for depression is Zoloft.[15] Yet, Zoloft is not approved for depression by the FDA. Indeed, in two studies that have been done of Zoloft for depressed children, the drug failed to be better than a placebo (dummy) pill.[16] When as much as 89 percent of antidepressants for children are off-label, this raises serious concerns since the FDA has now acknowledged that the drugs can make children suicidal.

When the British MHRA began virtually banning many antidepressants for children, the FDA had its internal reviewer, Andrew Mosholder, analyze the pharmaceutical company data on children taking the drugs. When Mosholder's analysis produced results similar to the British, the FDA suppressed his report in early 2004 and commissioned researchers at Columbia University to reanalyze the data once again. The Columbia reanalysis essentially replicated Mosholder's. In his report, Dr. Mosholder recommended "a risk management strategy directed at discouraging off-label pediatric use of antidepressant drugs, particularly the use of drugs other than Prozac in the treatment of pediatric MDD [major depression]."[17] After the Columbia reclassification essentially reproduced his results, Dr. Mosholder wrote that the results of the "Columbia University reclassification do not materially affect the recommendations

I made previously."[18] While the FDA's October 2004 black box warning that antidepressants can make children and adolescents suicidal is a major step forward, critics charge that it will still not do enough to protect American children, especially the vast majority of children receiving the drugs off-label, that is, for uses not approved by the FDA.

The controversy over children being prescribed antidepressants is not likely to be resolved in the near future, particularly because of the concerns that have been raised about the FDA, and conflicts of interest among academic researchers who work closely with the pharmaceutical industry. Concerned parents may want to read my earlier book, *Prozac Backlash: Overcoming the Dangers of Prozac, Zoloft, Paxil, and Other Antidepressants with Safe, Effective Alternatives. Prozac Backlash* describes all the side effects of the drugs, including how they can make patients suicidal; it examines the shortcomings in how the drugs are tested in children and adolescents to win FDA approval; and it discusses when drug treatment is a reasonable step to take as part of comprehensive psychiatric treatment versus when drug treatment is not appropriate.

Afterword

This book should never have needed to be written. When Paxil was introduced, GlaxoSmithKline reported that withdrawal reactions are "rare" with the new drug, which became a multibillion-dollar-a-year best seller.[1] When Zoloft was introduced, Pfizer made a similar claim that withdrawal reactions are "rare" with its best selling drug.[2] For perspective, keep in mind that officially the pharmaceutical industry itself defines rare side effects as occurring in less than one patient in a thousand, or .01 percent.[3] Paxil and Zoloft have since been shown to cause withdrawal reactions not in .01 percent but in 66 percent and 60 percent of patients, respectively.[4] How could pharmaceutical companies with their vast scientific and financial resources have been so wrong? How could companies miss withdrawal reactions that occur in 66 and 60 percent of patients so egregiously that they claimed they occurred in only 0.01 percent of patients?

When pharmaceutical companies test new antidepressants to win FDA approval, withdrawal reactions are typically not evaluated. The studies usually only last six to eight weeks, a remarkable fact given that patients subsequently take the drugs for years, even decades.[5] At the end of the six to eight weeks, the studies are over when the patients take their last dose. Since the studies are over, withdrawal symptoms are not assessed after the patients stop taking the drugs. This is sometimes referred to as the "Don't ask and you won't know" approach to evaluating—or, more accurately, not evaluating—side effects. That is how the companies were able to declare that withdrawal side effects rarely occur in patients. Elsewhere in the fine print of their official information on the drugs, the pharmaceutical companies note that dependence has "not been systematically studied."[6]

Why would pharmaceutical companies not want their drugs to be associated with withdrawal reactions? The answer is: Withdrawal implies dependence and addiction. In fact, in the modern era virtually all blockbuster psychiatric drugs have fallen on the sword of withdrawal, dependence, and addiction, along with other serious side effects. The drugs include Valium-type antianxiety agents, barbiturates, amphetamines, narcotics, and cocaine (originally a popular prescription drug, as described below). With Valium-type antianxiety agents, the last best sellers prior to today's best-selling antidepressants, by the 1990s pharmaceutical companies and the profession had learned the general principle that psychiatric drugs with shorter half-lives cause worse withdrawal and dependence. Withdrawal, dependence, and addiction have been *the* side effect that has plagued blockbuster psychiatric drugs. Why did we have to spend over a decade relearning this with today's antidepressants while countless patients and their families suffered?

Of the earlier classes of popular psychiatric drugs, today's antidepressants are most closely related to cocaine. A little over a hundred years ago, cocaine was the first prescription antidepressant of the modern era.[7] In the late 1800s and early 1900s, cocaine was the most popular prescription medication in Europe, prescribed for everything from depression to shyness, just as today's antidepressants are. At the turn of the century, Freud wrote three famous "cocaine papers" extolling cocaine's benefits.[8] At the height of its popularity, cocaine was the essential ingredient in Coca-Cola, which is named after cocaine.[9] It took pharmaceutical companies decades to acknowledge cocaine's dangerous side effects, including severe withdrawal reactions and addiction. Only afterwards did caffeine replace cocaine in Coca-Cola.

Surprisingly, cocaine is a "reuptake inhibitor" that increases the signals of three "feel good" neurotransmitters, or chemical signals, in the brain: serotonin, dopamine, and noradrenalin, the form of adrenalin found in the brain.[10] I say surprisingly, because as seen in Table A.1, today's popular antidepressants are promoted as also increasing one or more of these closely related "feel good" signals. Indeed, most of today's

Table A.1 COMPARISON OF COCAINE WITH TODAY'S ANTIDEPRESSANTS

		Neurotransmitters Boosted		
		Serotonin	Noradrenalin	Dopamine
	Cocaine	✓	✓	✓
SSRIs	Prozac	✓		
	Zoloft	✓		✓
	Paxil	✓		
	Luvox	✓		
	Celexa	✓		
	Lexapro	✓		
SNRIs	Effexor	✓	✓	
	Cymbalta	✓	✓	
	Serzone	✓	✓	
Other	Wellbutrin			✓
	Remeron	✓	✓	
	"Cocktail" of Wellbutrin and an SSRI	✓		✓
	"Cocktail" of Wellbutrin and an SNRI, or Remeron	✓	✓	✓

Most of today's antidepressants boost serotonin, noradrenalin, and/or dopamine by the same principal mechanism as cocaine (i.e., reuptake inhibition)—including all of the SSRIs, Effexor, Cymbalta, and Wellbutrin.

antidepressants boost these signals by the same principle mechanism as cocaine. Like cocaine they are "reuptake inhibitors." The first of today's popular antidepressants, Prozac, boosts serotonin and is marketed as a selective serotonin reuptake inhibitor, or SSRI.[11] The next one, Zoloft, boosts serotonin and dopamine.[12] Effexor boosts serotonin and noradrenalin; it is marketed as a serotonin and noradrenalin reuptake inhibitor, or SNRI.[13] Wellbutrin boosts dopamine.[14] Many patients are prescribed "cocktails" of two or three antidepressants, such as Effexor and Wellbutrin, which together boost all three neurotransmitters, much

The Antidepressant Solution

like cocaine. All of the drugs in Table A.1 have secondary effects on other neurotransmitters that are not fully understood. None of the drugs are identical to one another but they are closely related in their mechanisms of action and effects on brain chemicals.

According to *Goodman & Gilman's The Pharmacological Basis of Therapeutics,* the leading medical textbook of pharmacology, when cocaine is taken orally at doses that are not excessive (i.e., at doses given when it was legally prescribed), it produces increased energy, alertness, ability to concentrate, self-confidence, and a sense of well-being, much like today's antidepressants.[15] The overstimulating, "high" effects associated with cocaine occur when it is *abused* in high doses, especially when taken via routes of administration more rapid than oral administration— that is, via snorting or intravenous injection. The cravings associated with cocaine occur when it is abused in these illicit ways. When taken at prescription doses, cocaine did not cause the cravings seen in patients who abuse the drug but it did cause withdrawal reactions if stopped abruptly.

If cocaine were discovered today and promoted as a new antidepressant, it would likely be marketed as a serotonin, noradrenalin, and dopamine reuptake inhibitor, or SNDRI. Since this is a mouthful, cocaine would probably be promoted as a "super neurotransmitter" reuptake inhibitor, because it boosts all three "feel good" chemicals in the brain. In fact, "new" antidepressants that boost all three signals are already in the pipeline.[16] They are on the cutting edge of research and development of "new" antidepressants. Indeed, they have already been named "super neurotransmitter" reuptake inhibitors.[17] But, isn't this all too much like reinventing cocaine? How could the pharmaceutical industry have thought drugs this closely related to cocaine would not cause withdrawal and dependence?

Some fifteen years after today's popular antidepressants were first introduced, a book like this was necessary to set the record straight: to provide patients and doctors with the information they need on antidepressant withdrawal and dependence. Unfortunately, history is repeating itself in the way this side effect has been handled. The current attention being given to the serious side effects of today's antidepressants is appearing right on schedule, like clockwork in what I call a 10-20-30-year pattern typical of the side effects of popular psychiatric drugs.[18] Once new drugs are released to the market, the FDA lacks a systematic program for monitoring their side effects. Instead, the agency relies on spontaneous reports from doctors who are typically too busy to notify the FDA of all the side effects they see in patients.[19] Indeed, Dr. David Kessler, former head of the FDA and now dean of the Yale School of Medicine, has stated "only about 1 percent of serious events [side effects] are reported" to the agency.[20]

As a result, it often takes a decade before the most serious side effects of a new class of psychiatric drugs are identified. Because pharmaceutical companies have adamantly denied the side effects, it takes another decade for enough data to accumulate for the problems to be undeniable and for a number of patient advocates to be sounding the alarm. Yet a third decade typically elapses before the slow bureaucracies of regulatory agencies and professional organizations act to change treatment guidelines and prescribing patterns. By the time this 10-20-30-year pattern plays itself out, what were once "new" drugs have become old, their patents have expired, and they are no longer profitable. By this time, the pharmaceutical companies have abandoned the drugs and moved on to newly patented, more profitable ones that can be promoted as "safer" largely because their side effects are unknown. Indeed, in some instances the companies turn on their old drugs whose patents have expired, helping to discredit them to pave the way for new ones. The attention now being focused on the side effects of today's antidepressants is right on schedule: These drugs have been on the market a little over fifteen years, the patents on several of them have already expired, and the pharmaceutical industry has relaxed its once fierce defense of them.

Exceptions to this rule occur when one or two antidepressants cause a side effect less frequently. In some instances, the manufacturers of these drugs will fund and publicize studies of the side effect of a competing company's drug in an effort to gain market share for its own drug. For example, in the mid-1990s, the manufacturers of Wellbutrin and Serzone funded studies of antidepressant-induced sexual side effects, comparing their drugs to SSRIs like Prozac and Zoloft.[21] The studies corroborated the high incidence of sexual side effects found in patients taking SSRIs, some 60 percent of patients, and claimed an advantage for Wellbutrin and Serzone. Company-funded researchers even held a press conference to announce the results.[22] The resulting publicity was largely responsible for alerting doctors and the public to the high incidence of sexual side effects in patients on SSRI-type antidepressants.[23] Unfortunately, many other serious side effects of antidepressants do not receive this kind of careful study and publicity when no one drug has such a clear advantage. Under these circumstances, no company is motivated to fund the necessary studies to demonstrate and publicize its advantage. That such politics and marketing play a large role in what side effects we have good data on is regrettable.

In the case of antidepressant withdrawal reactions, Prozac has an advantage. In a large-scale, systematic study of over 200 patients, 14 percent of patients stopping Prozac had withdrawal reactions.[24] By contrast, 66 percent of patients stopping Paxil and 60 percent of patients stopping Zoloft experienced withdrawal reactions. Not surprisingly, Eli Lilly is the company that funded the study comparing its own drug Prozac to competitors Paxil and Zoloft. The study took place in the mid-1990s as sales of Paxil and Zoloft threatened to eclipse Prozac sales. In this effort Lilly walked a tightrope: While "educating" doctors about the advantages of Prozac, Lilly had to avoid calling unwanted attention to the phenomenon of antidepressant withdrawal, with its serious implication— that is, dependence—for all antidepressants. Negotiating this tricky balance, Lilly is also the company that funded the campaign to rename antidepressant withdrawal reactions "antidepressant discontinuation syndrome."[25] In a carefully orchestrated effort, the Lilly-funded campaign deflected attention away from the more serious implications of antidepressant withdrawal reactions while Prozac gained the advantage over its competitors on this particular side effect.[26]

Prozac's advantage in the Lilly-funded study on withdrawal has been controversial.[27] In the study, patients stopped their antidepressants abruptly for five to eight days and were systematically monitored for withdrawal side effects. Systematic monitoring means a checklist of antidepressant withdrawal symptoms was used to inquire in detail about withdrawal reactions. Repeated studies have found that less systematic, more open-ended questions or not asking at all (relying on spontaneous reports) detect much lower rates of a side effect.[28] Systematic monitoring is essential to determining the true incidence of side effects. But because of Prozac's long half-life, withdrawal reactions typically do not appear within five to eight days. Rather, they take two to three weeks or more. Critics charge that the design of the Lilly-sponsored study was biased in Prozac's favor.[29]

Lilly conducted a separate study that addresses the issue.[30] In this study, patients stopped Prozac and were monitored for six weeks. However, when one examines the study closely, one discovers that patients were not systematically monitored for withdrawal symptoms. Instead of using a checklist to inquire about specific symptoms, patients were asked open-ended questions about "general well-being and problems with medication."[31] In other words, Prozac was not held to the same standard that Paxil and Zoloft had been in the withdrawal study utilizing the five-to-eight-day time frame.

To conduct and publish such studies, pharmaceutical companies work closely with industry-friendly academic psychiatrists. Jerrold Rosenbaum, professor of psychiatry at Harvard Medical School and chief of psychiatry at Massachusetts General Hospital, conducted the key study for Eli Lilly that compared Prozac to Paxil and Zoloft with a five-to-eight-day time frame.[32] Rosenbaum also coauthored the study specifically looking at Prozac withdrawal that did not hold Lilly's drug to the same standard to which its competitors were held.[33] And, Rosenbaum was a key player in the Lilly-funded campaign to replace the term "antidepressant withdrawal" with "antidepressant discontinuation syndrome."[34] Indeed, in a roundtable discussion published in 1997, Rosenbaum announced the full scope of Lilly's ambitious project to rename the phenomenon and study their drug in comparison with others.[35]

Rosenbaum is no stranger to controversy over his relationship with Eli Lilly and Prozac. He played a pivotal role in the controversy over the suicidal effects of today's antidepressants when the controversy first exploded in the media in the early 1990s.[36] At the time, only Prozac, the first of today's antidepressants, was on the market. As the controversy raged, Rosenbaum came to Prozac's defense in 1991, publishing *the* definitive study in the *Journal of Clinical Psychiatry* insisting Prozac does not make adults suicidal.[37] In the study, Rosenbaum compared data on Prozac with data on earlier classes of antidepressants, claiming that his statistical analysis showed that Prozac does not cause higher rates of suicidality. Rosenbaum's study was hugely influential in large part because he appeared to be an academic psychiatrist independent of Eli Lilly. Similar defenses of Prozac published by in-house Eli Lilly psychiatrists did not have the same impact.[38] But a May 7, 2000 *Boston Globe* exposé revealed that Rosenbaum's "1991 study on Prozac and suicide [has been] criticized by at least two sets of researchers as well as the FDA."[39] The critiques the *Boston Globe* was referring to, including the one by the FDA, argued Rosenbaum got his statistics wrong: his own data show that Prozac is associated with about a threefold greater incidence of suicidality than older, comparison antidepressants, the critics said.[40] What is more, the *Boston Globe* revealed that Rosenbaum had a "cozy" relationship advising Eli Lilly's marketing department on Prozac since "before

Prozac was launched," that is, before it was introduced to the market in the late 1980s. Rosenbaum did not reveal his behind-the-scenes ties to Lilly's marketing department in his influential 1991 study on Prozac-induced suicidality. Rosenbaum's was the key study silencing the controversy for almost a decade.[41] This is the same side effect in adults that has reemerged in recent years because of newly revealed studies showing that children and adolescents become suicidal on many of today's antidepressants. In the meantime, pharmaceutical companies have paid scores of secret settlements in lawsuits involving antidepressant-induced suicides and murder-suicides of adults and children. For Rosenbaum not to have divulged his behind-the-scenes relationship with Lilly's marketing department when he was apparently wrong in his influential 1991 study is deeply troubling.

If one compares Rosenbaum's statements on antidepressant withdrawal reactions published in medical journals with his statements in the general media aimed at the public, one can see him walking the same tightrope Eli Lilly has walked on this side effect. In his large-scale, systematic study published in *Biological Psychiatry,* Rosenbaum calls doctors' attention to the high rates of withdrawal reactions with antidepressants that have short half-lives: 66 percent of patients with Paxil and 60 percent with Zoloft.[42] He cites numerous other reports of withdrawal reactions including one conducted by the British MHRA in which 57 percent of patients who experienced Paxil withdrawal had to restart the drug because of moderately severe or severe withdrawal reactions.[43] Sounding the alarm in an article in the *Journal of Clinical Psychiatry,* Rosenbaum says that withdrawal symptoms "have an adverse effect on *many* patients' quality of life and have led to missed work days, lower productivity, and higher medical costs. In one study, 5 of 14 patients who discontinued Luvox treatment took at least 1 day off from work, and 3 sought medical attention locally. Another patient was confined to bed and absent from work for 3 days because of severe dizziness associated with Paxil discontinuation [emphasis added]."[44] Rosenbaum points out that in patients stopping Effexor withdrawal reactions "occur *dramatically and commonly* [emphasis added]."[45] Regarding how little many doctors know about antidepressant withdrawal reactions, Rosenbaum cautions: "*many often* fail to recognize and/or diagnose" withdrawal reactions [emphasis added].[46] When this happens, antidepressant withdrawal symptoms can be "misdiagnosed as depressive relapse and, as a result, the patient may [needlessly] resume antidepressant treatment."

Rosenbaum concludes that "gradual tapering is necessary for all serotonin reuptake inhibitors (SRIs) except Prozac."[47]

Despite the antidepressant withdrawal alarm he sounds in medical journals while calling attention to Prozac's advantage, when Rosenbaum is quoted in the general media one hears a somewhat different story. In April 2003, *Glamour* magazine ran an article on Paxil withdrawal entitled "Addicted to Antidepressants?" Interviewed in the *Glamour* article, Rosenbaum says that only about "one in 10 patients will experience problems if the drug [Paxil] is abruptly discontinued."[48] Why would Rosenbaum say that only 10 percent of patients stopping Paxil abruptly experience "problems" when he published the definitive study demonstrating that 66 percent experience withdrawal reactions? What did he mean by "problems" when he cited this low number that minimizes the impact of antidepressant withdrawal reactions? This was not an isolated incident; Rosenbaum has repeatedly made statements downplaying the issue to the public in the general media. Rosenbaum was quoted in a May 25, 2004 article in the *New York Times* entitled, "The Consumer: How to Stop Depression Medications."[49] He told the *New York Times* that "studies suggest that only 10 to 20 percent of patients have significant problems" with antidepressant withdrawal reactions. Whereas in medical journals Rosenbaum warns of the dangers of withdrawal reactions being misdiagnosed as depressive relapse, the *Times* article emphasizes Rosenbaum cautioning: "Just because you're stopping a drug doesn't mean you don't need it."

Internal GlaxoSmithKline documents reveal that the manufacturer of Paxil lost no time organizing a response to Lilly. A May 1, 1997 GlaxoSmithKline memo states: "Lilly has initiated a new campaign focused on discontinuation symptoms associated with cessation of SSRI" antidepressants.[50] Another report argues: Lilly has created a "marketing campaign focusing on the higher incidence of withdrawal symptoms associated with Paxil compared to Prozac" because "Lilly has seen a precipitous drop in their market share over the past two years while Paxil market share has been soaring."[51] And a June 5, 1997 memo from GlaxoSmithKline's public relations firm, Ruder Finn, describes the steps it is taking for the pharmaceutical giant to refute "what Rosenbaum et al. state or allege."[52]

The Ruder Finn memo provides a rare glimpse into how the public relations firms of pharmaceutical behemoths seek to influence the practice of medicine behind the scenes. The Ruder Finn memo states that the public relations firm has ghostwritten two proposed responses to Rosenbaum and his colleagues' articles. The memo suggests the Glaxo-SmithKline-friendly psychiatrists who will author the responses. The memo proposes that one of the pieces will be authored by Dr. Bruce Pollock, professor of psychiatry at the University of Pittsburgh School of Medicine. Four months later, Dr. Pollock published a response to Rosenbaum and his colleagues' articles in the October 1998 issue of the *Journal of Clinical Psychiatry*.[53] Pollock's published piece is expanded and elaborated in more formal, academic language. But it raises many of the same points and follows much the same line of arguments as Ruder Finn's. While the timing of Pollock's published piece and Ruder Finn's could be a coincidence, the Ruder Finn memo provides direct evidence of pharmaceutical company public relations firms seeking to influence academic publications authored in the name of seemingly independent psychiatrists. Pollock's published piece does not mention his apparent behind-the-scenes relationship with GlaxoSmithKline or Ruder Finn. In fact, Pollock has been a consultant to GlaxoSmithKline.[54] He has also received grant research money, been paid honoraria, and been a member of the company's speakers bureau or advisory boards.

The Ruder Finn memo describes a second ghostwritten piece on the same subject to be authored by yet another GlaxoSmithKline-friendly psychiatrist. In a comical vein the memo notes that the footnotes in the two pieces are "the same" and "complete duplication will look fishy if we decide to submit both" for publication. "Are there other references we could draw on for various drugs?" the memo asks, adding, "At the very least we can't have the references appear in the same order." Presumably, by "fishy" Ruder Finn meant that the duplicate footnotes in the same order might be a giveaway that the two pieces originated from the same source, in this instance a pharmaceutical company's public relations firm ghostwriting the original versions. It appears the second piece was not submitted for publication, which may be how Ruder Finn solved the footnote problem.

In the late 1990s, GlaxoSmithKline went to considerable effort to train its sales force in how to "educate" doctors about the growing concerns of Paxil withdrawal. Repeated studies have shown that pharmaceutical company sales representatives have enormous influence over doctors who rely on them for up-to-date information. GlaxoSmithKline instructed its sales representatives that if doctors said, "I won't use Paxil because of withdrawal symptoms," the sales reps should "minimize" the concern by assuring doctors that discontinuation symptoms are "generally mild," "transient," and "infrequent." Indeed, despite a confidential, internal company report describing studies indicating as many as 62 percent of people stopping Paxil developed withdrawal symptoms that in some cases could be "severe" and "disabling," a 1997 GlaxoSmithKline "Business Plan Guide" told its sales force to reassure doctors that Paxil withdrawal only occurs in "two in 1,000 patients or 0.2%."[55] (Note that the guide had the math wrong: two in 1,000 patients is 0.002 percent.) The guide told GlaxoSmithKline sales representatives that "all of the SSRIs exhibit similar rates of discontinuation symptoms" even though numerous reports published by 1997 had established that this is not the case.[56] The guide instructs sales reps on how to speak differently about Paxil to family doctors versus psychiatrists, given their different expertise.

Another sales training guide features Dr. Bruce Pollock's response to the Eli Lilly campaign as "an effective tool for addressing discontinuation."[57] The response, says the guide, is "authored by Bruce Pollack, M.D. in the *Journal of Clinical Psychiatry* October 1998." It "is a great resource for addressing the issue of discontinuation [with doctors]. Dr. Pollack clarifies that discontinuation symptoms have been reported to occur with *all* SSRIs with onset and duration mediated by drug half-life [with no mention of different frequencies mediated by half-life]. Most importantly, he balances the risk benefit of a short vs. long half-life. . . . You may order reprints of the Pollack" response "electronically" to give to doctors. (Note that Pollock's name is misspelled in the guide.) The guide did not divulge to GlaxoSmithKline's representatives that the pharmaceutical giant's public relations firm, Ruder Finn, had ghostwritten a proposed piece the firm wanted Dr. Pollock to publish.

The Business Plan Guide explains that part of GlaxoSmithKline's strategy is to "increase support of Paxil by thought leaders in psychiatry and other opinion leaders to positively impact sales in the institutions and the community."[58] Pharmaceutical companies use the terms "thought leaders" and "opinion leaders" to refer to psychiatrists they work closely with to promote their drugs. "Opinion leaders" aptly describes the influence these doctors exert on the medical community, aided by the pharmaceutical industry's vast resources and even, in some instances, by ghostwriting assistance publishing influential papers in academic journals.

Another educational program for GlaxoSmithKline's sales reps admits explicitly that " 'withdrawal syndrome' is a class effect that can occur when an SSRI is stopped abruptly," but urges sales representatives that when talking to doctors "instead of 'withdrawal syndrome' . . . try to refer to this phenomenon as 'discontinuation symptoms' " because withdrawal syndrome "implies addiction properties."[59] In fact, one confidential, internal GlaxoSmithKline "Safety Review of [Paxil] Discontinuation Symptoms" describes patients abusing the drug.[60] One patient "crushed tablets and injected a 'very chalky' mixture concocted from a suspension of the [Paxil] powder." Another took "30 tablets of Paxil in two doses over a two-day period "in order to obtain a 'buzz.' " Still another GlaxoSmithKline guide coaches sales representatives that when talking to doctors about Paxil withdrawal "don't focus on the incidence," instead "emphasize the benign nature and good clinical practice (to taper)."[61]

A transmittal memo that accompanied one confidential, internal GlaxoSmithKline report on "Paxil and the incidence of discontinuation symptoms" cautions: "Please note that this information is for in-house use only and is not to be passed to regulatory authorities [such as the FDA], external investigators, or clinicians [i.e. practicing doctors]."[62] Another GlaxoSmithKline guide raises the question "Discontinuation: Why this is an issue." It answers: "Paxil sales to end [of] Sept[ember] 1997] already exceed $1 BILLION."[63] The "$1 BILLION" is in large, bold letters. Beneath the bold headline is artwork showing a huge moneybag with a dollar sign emblazoned on it.

One internal GlaxoSmithKline memo to the "Paxil selling team" on "discontinuation syndrome[s]" ends with a particularly offensive cartoon of a woman patient. The headline of the cartoon says: "Let's face it in the end. The only thing the anxious and agitated patient will be saying is 'Where's my Paxil!!!!!!' "[64] The cartoon depicts a hysterical-looking woman sitting at her desk, screaming at the top of her lungs, throwing her hands up, and tossing all her papers into the air while yelling, "Where's my Paxil!!!!!!" The woman's mouth is stretched open so exaggeratedly that it obliterates most of the rest of her face. The cartoon is demeaning to all patients but particularly to women, who are prescribed the majority of antidepressants. Most people would be surprised by such a derogatory attitude toward patients and by such a carefully orchestrated effort that misleads doctors and patients. The cruel irony is that patients can be distraught enough to ask, "Where's my Paxil?" when they are in severe Paxil withdrawal. The cartoon could be viewed as depicting patients hooked on the prescription drug.

For over a decade "cozy" relationships have flourished between pharmaceutical companies and a small coterie of academic psychiatrists who can each make millions consulting to the companies, advising their marketing departments, doing research with the companies, and publishing papers that can be ghostwritten by the companies.[65] When pharmaceutical companies design research so that it is biased in favor of their drugs or when they selectively publish only those results that are favorable to their drugs, they are misleading practicing physicians who need complete, unbiased information to exercise their professional judgment in the best interest of patients. Academic psychiatrists who make millions of dollars consulting to the companies are not truly independent when they extol the companies' drugs to the public. But this is not obvious to the public and the media when the doctors and the companies have not divulged the extent of these behind-the-scenes relationships.

Unfortunately, in the last decade deceptive practices have become routine in the researching, publishing, and marketing of psychiatric drugs, making it extremely difficult for patients and practicing physicians to get accurate, balanced information.[66] Now, with the FDA's warnings that antidepressants may make children and adults suicidal and the British MHRA's virtually banning many antidepressants for children, these practices are coming under closer scrutiny. Eliot Spitzer, the attorney general of New York, sued GlaxoSmithKline for fraud for withholding data from its studies of children taking Paxil.[67] GlaxoSmithKline settled the suit before it went to trial. Pfizer paid a $430 million settlement in a lawsuit involving deceptive marketing of its psychiatric drug Neurontin.[68] These are major advances for patients and patient advocates, especially since the FDA has not adequately held pharmaceutical companies and their appointed "opinion leaders" accountable.

Indeed, the FDA has contributed significantly to the problem of both of the antidepressant side effects currently receiving widespread attention: withdrawal reactions and the drugs making patients suicidal. In the case of the drugs making patients suicidal, the FDA learned of this side effect more than a decade ago, in the early 1990s, shortly after Prozac was introduced.[69] The FDA convened an advisory panel of nine experts and held a hearing on the issue in September 1991 because of widespread public and professional concern.[70] Unfortunately, the committee was rife with conflicts of interest. The FDA had to waive its own standards for conflicts of interest for five of the nine committee members because of their ties to the pharmaceutical industry.[71] Despite the many conflicts of interest, one-third of the committee members voted for a warning in 1991, over a decade ago![72] What is more, if one reads the transcript of the hearing, the FDA and its advisory committee repeatedly called for more research.

In fact, at the height of the controversy in the early 1990s, the FDA and Eli Lilly agreed to a large-scale, systematic study of antidepressant-induced suicidality to better characterize and understand the phenomenon.[73] However, once the media attention to the problem died down, the research was never done.[74] When the issue resurfaced in the media in 2003 after the British MHRA all but banned most SSRIs for children and adolescents because of this side effect, many observers found the FDA's calls for more research an outrage coming more than a decade after the agency had failed to follow through with research it knew was needed all along.[75] When the FDA's own in-house expert, Dr. Andrew Mosholder, reviewed the data on children and adolescents, he came to conclusions similar to the British.[76] But, the FDA muzzled Mosholder, suppressed his report, and spent months having researchers at Columbia University reanalyze the data. The Columbia researchers reached essentially the same conclusions that Mosholder and the British had.[77] The FDA's handling of the antidepressant scandal has become the subject of a congressional investigation.[78]

With regard to antidepressant withdrawal reactions, the FDA has not demanded that pharmaceutical companies assess withdrawal symptoms adequately when they test new antidepressants for FDA approval. The FDA knew or should have known from experience with earlier classes of psychiatric drugs that antidepressants with short and ultra-short half-lives would inevitably cause withdrawal and dependence. Since withdrawal reactions with today's antidepressants have come to the attention of doctors and the public, the FDA has allowed pharmaceutical companies to call withdrawal reactions antidepressant "discontinuation" symptoms in their official information on the drugs. Withdrawal reactions are still listed as "rare" side effects of drugs like Paxil and Effexor in the companies' official information.[79] For details on withdrawal symptoms, one needs to know to look elsewhere under antidepressant "discontinuation," despite the fact that leading psychiatric textbooks and academic papers describe "antidepressant discontinuation syndromes" and "antidepressant withdrawal reactions" as one and the same.[80] The FDA approves the companies' official information on the drugs word-for-word and lets them get away with this semantic gamesmanship at the expense of patients and doctors. Hiding behind the term "antidepressant discontinuation syndrome," the industry has repeatedly denied that today's antidepressants cause withdrawal reactions. The companies have promoted antidepressants as "non habit-forming," "not associated with dependence or addiction," and causing "mild, usually temporary, side effects" with FDA approval.[81] Indeed, when a patient advocacy lawsuit convinced a California judge to ban such deceptive advertising, the FDA intervened on behalf of the pharmaceutical industry, claiming the judge had no jurisdiction.[82] The FDA's mandate is to protect consumers, not drug company profits. The FDA's actions are another example of the unprecedented behind-the-scenes political power wielded today by the pharmaceutical industry lobby. In addition to political pressure on the FDA, critics point to lucrative pharmaceutical company consulting contracts awarded to FDA officials while they are working at the agency and especially after they leave it.[83]

Another federal agency expected to be an objective, impartial protector of the public interest is the National Institutes of Health, NIH. Unfortunately, in recent years the NIH, too, has been rocked by scandal: many of its top officials have had lucrative consulting contracts with pharmaceutical companies. In December 2003, a *Los Angeles Times* exposé revealed that top NIH scientists received hundreds of thousands of dollars—in at least one instance over a million dollars—in consulting fees from pharmaceutical companies.[84] In some instances, NIH department heads received behind-the-scenes consulting fees while their departments were providing the companies with millions of taxpayer dollars in NIH research grants. The FDA's and NIH's pro-industry stances have left the American public with inadequate consumer protection and patient advocacy in the face of pharmaceutical company political clout.

Dr. Marcia Angell, former editor-in-chief of the *New England Journal of Medicine* and a senior lecturer in social medicine at Harvard Medical School, describes the pharmaceutical industry's pervasive influence over academic medicine, the FDA, and NIH as examples of the industry's ability to "co-opt every institution that might stand in its way."[85] As one of the most profitable industries in the country, the pharmaceutical industry is awash with money with which to buy influence. Pharmaceutical companies defend their price gouging and outrageous profits as necessary to support their research and development activities. But Angell points out that this is not true: The pharmaceutical industry's spending on research and development is dwarfed by its spending on marketing and advertising campaigns. The industry spends more than a third of its revenues on marketing, more than two and a half times what it spends on research and development. Because heavy advertising and marketing substantially increase the costs of drugs, costs that are ultimately paid for by health insurance, the pharmaceutical industry's exorbitant promotion of its drugs drains the financially strapped health care system.

Public opinion is turning against the pharmaceutical industry. Much of the American public is disillusioned with the industry's price gouging and the avalanche of revelations of deceptive marketing and fraud. A July 2004 Harris poll surveying public opinion on a variety of major industries found that people ranked pharmaceutical companies among the lowest.[86] The pharmaceutical industry shares its low status with the tobacco industry and managed care health insurance companies. We have all been reluctant to come to this conclusion. Pharmaceutical companies and medications are an essential part of the health care system. Countless patients benefit from medication of many different kinds. But the revelations of price gouging, exorbitant profits, and deceptive practices have forced a reluctant public to lower its opinion of pharmaceutical companies. Unfortunately, psychiatry is particularly vulnerable to the pharmaceutical industry's deceptive practices when researching and marketing drugs. This is because the diagnosis of psychiatric conditions and the response to psychiatric medication is so subjective and therefore so easily manipulated.[87]

Practicing doctors do not want to mislead patients. Most doctors want to make decisions in the best interests of their patients. Not surprisingly, doctors are upset to discover that pharmaceutical companies and the "expert" doctors who work closely with the industry have misled them. Doctors and patients need to take medicine back from the pharmaceutical industry and its appointed "experts." An independent FDA committed to consumer advocacy and protection would seem a reasonable expectation for a publicly funded government agency.

To make amends for misleading patients and doctors about antidepressant withdrawal and dependence, at a minimum, pharmaceutical companies should be required to:

- Make pills available in many more milligram sizes to facilitate tapering today's antidepressants
- Conduct a well-funded campaign to educate doctors and the public about antidepressant withdrawal, including television, newspaper, and magazine advertisements

- Abandon the misleading term "antidepressant discontinuation syndrome" for the straightforward term "antidepressant withdrawal reaction" in all descriptions of the phenomenon
- Include warning labels on patients' antidepressant prescription bottles that the drugs can cause severe withdrawal reactions, should not be stopped abruptly, and need to be taken every day exactly as prescribed to avoid withdrawal reactions that might be confused with a worsening of the patient's underlying psychiatric condition
- When testing all future antidepressants for FDA approval, systematically monitor and accurately report the percentage of patients who have withdrawal reactions
- Publish all psychiatric drug studies, not just those favorable to the companies' marketing interests

For most of this book I have avoided the murky politics of why doctors and patients do not know more about antidepressant withdrawal and dependence. Instead, I treated withdrawal and dependence as problems we need to solve in as straightforward a fashion as possible. But in this Afterword, I have given you a glimpse into the darker side of why doctors and patients know so little about antidepressant withdrawal and dependence.

As you finish reading this book, you will probably come to a decision with your doctor about whether you are ready to try tapering off your antidepressant. If you embark on a tapering program, take the time to wean off the drug safely and comfortably. If you start the taper from a modest dose and have little or no withdrawal symptoms, you may complete the taper in less than two months. On the other hand, if you start from a higher dose or have severe withdrawal reactions, the taper may take you many more months.

Once you stop taking the drug completely, be sure to stay in touch with your doctor and therapist. Patients should be encouraged to continue to see their doctor and therapist at least once a month in the initial months after stopping an antidepressant altogether. All too often, patients being treated in HMOs or other managed care settings get the impression that they are only entitled to the doctor's attention if they are on medication. Instead, they should be encouraged to see their doctor as regularly when they are off the drugs as they did when they were on them, at least for a while, to be sure they do fine off the drugs.

Many patients who have recently finished antidepressant tapering programs panic the first time they have a bad day, fearing their depression has returned. But a bad day is not the same thing as clinical depression. Ask yourself: "Did I have bad days when I was on an antidepressant?" Most people find the answer is "Yes." A supportive doctor can help you maintain perspective and get through the transition back to living medication-free.

Appendix 1

DAILY CHECKLIST OF ANTIDEPRESSANT WITHDRAWAL SYMPTOMS

The 5-Step Antidepressant Tapering Program

Name: _____   Antidepressant: _____

Day: _____ *(1, 2, 3, etc. since last dosage reduction)* Date: _____ Day of week: _____

Dose prior to this reduction: _____ mg/day   New dose: _____ mg/day

PSYCHIATRIC SYMPTOMS	✓	MEDICAL SYMPTOMS	✓
That Mimic Depression		*That Mimic the Flu*	
1. Crying spells		29. Flu-like aches and pains	
2. Worsened mood		30. Fever	
3. Low energy (fatigue, lethargy, malaise)		31. Sweats	
4. Trouble concentrating		32. Chills	
5. Insomnia or trouble sleeping		33. Runny nose	
6. Change in appetite		34. Sore eyes	
7. Suicidal thoughts			
8. Suicide attempts		*That Mimic Gastroenteritis*	
		35. Nausea	
That Mimic Anxiety Disorders		36. Vomiting	
9. Anxious, nervous, tense		37. Diarrhea	
10. Panic attacks (racing heart, breathless)		38. Abdominal pain or cramps	
11. Chest pain		39. Stomach bloating	
12. Trembling, jittery, or shaking			
		Dizziness	
Irritability and Aggression		40. Disequilibrium	
13. Irritability		41. Spinning, swaying, lightheaded	
14. Agitation (restlessness, hyperactivity)		42. Hung over or waterlogged feeling	
15. Impulsivity		43. Unsteady gait, poor coordination	
16. Aggressiveness		44. Motion sickness	
17. Self-harm			
18. Homicidal thoughts or urges		*Headache*	
		45. Headache	
Confusion and Memory Problems			
19. Confusion or cognitive difficulties		*Tremor*	
20. Memory problems or forgetfulness		46. Tremor	
Mood Swings		*Sensory Abnormalities*	
21. Elevated mood (feeling high)		47. Numbness, burning, or tingling	
22. Mood swings		48. Electric zap-like sensations in the brain	
23. Manic-like reactions		49. Electric shock-like sensations in the body	
		50. Abnormal visual sensations	
Hallucinations		51. Ringing or other noises in the ears	
24. Auditory hallucinations		52. Abnormal smells or tastes	
25. Visual hallucinations			
		Other	
Dissociation		53. Drooling or excessive saliva	
26. Feeling detached or unreal		54. Slurred speech	
		55. Blurred vision	
Other		56. Muscle cramps, stiffness, twitches	
27. Excessive or intense dreaming		57. Feeling of restless legs	
28. Nightmares		58. Uncontrollable twitching of mouth	

Global assessment of severity of withdrawal symptoms for the day

	None	Mild			Moderate				Severe		
	0	1	2	3	4	5	6	7	8	9	10
✓											

Copyright 2005 © Joseph Glenmullen, MD   www.antidepressantsolution.com

Appendix 2

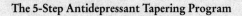

GRAPH OF AN ANTIDEPRESSANT WITHDRAWAL REACTION

The 5-Step Antidepressant Tapering Program

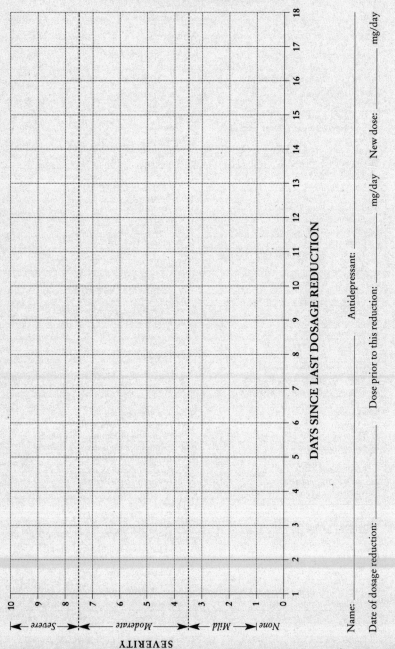

SEVERITY

None — Mild — Moderate — Severe

DAYS SINCE LAST DOSAGE REDUCTION

Antidepressant: _____

Dose prior to this reduction: _____ mg/day   New dose: _____ mg/day

Name: _____

Date of dosage reduction: _____

Appendix 3

Tapering Older Tricyclic and Heterocyclic Antidepressants

Tricyclic antidepressants were the most commonly prescribed antidepressants in the 1980s, before the introduction of Prozac, although they never achieved the popularity of today's best-selling antidepressants. Tricyclic antidepressants have irritating side effects like dry mouth, upset stomach, and lightheadedness that put a damper on their use. As a result, tricyclic antidepressants were only used when genuinely needed for moderate to severe depression, unlike today's best-selling antidepressants, which have been widely overprescribed to patients for a host of mild conditions.[1] Tricyclic antidepressants were almost exclusively prescribed by psychiatrists, whereas today's popular antidepressants are largely prescribed by family doctors. Today's best-selling antidepressants are no more effective than the older, tricyclic antidepressants; all antidepressants, new and old, are equally effective for depression.[2] Since the October 2004 update, the FDA's warnings that people may become suicidal on antidepressants also apply to these older drugs.

The name tricyclic refers to the three-ring structure of the original antidepressants in this class.[3] When some of the later additions to the group had more than three rings in their chemical structures, the technically more correct term "heterocyclic" antidepressants was introduced. Still, the group is popularly known by the original name tricyclic antidepressants, which is therefore the term I will use for the group.

Remarkably, most of the tricyclic antidepressants are still available, in generic and/or brand name form, as seen in Table App. 3.1.[4] Having been introduced in the 1950s, by the 1980s tricyclic antidepressants were routinely tapered because of withdrawal reactions.[5] Notice in the table that the tricyclic antidepressants are typically available in a much wider range of pill sizes than today's popular antidepressants, alleviating the need to cut pills into fragments and making it much easier to taper the drugs.

Table App 3.1 TRICYCLIC AND HETEROCYCLIC ANTIDEPRESSANTS

	Usual Therapeutic Dosage (mg/day)	Generic Pill Sizes (mg)	Brand Name Pill Sizes (mg)
Imipramine	100–300	10, 25, 50	*Tofranil*—10, 25, 50, 75, 100, 125, 150 *Tofranil PM*—75, 100, 125, 150
Desipramine	100–300	25, 50, 100	*Norpramin*—10, 25, 50, 75, 100, 150
Trimipramine	100–300	Not available	*Surmontil*—25, 50, 100
Clomipramine	100–300	25, 50, 75	*Anafranil*—25, 50, 75
Doxepin	100–300	10, 25, 50, 75, 100, 150	*Sinequan*—10, 25, 50, 75, 100, 150, liquid
Maprotiline	100–300	25, 50, 75	*Ludiomil*—Brand name no longer available
Nortriptyline	50–150	10, 25, 50, 75, liquid	*Pamelor*—10, 25, 50, 75, liquid *Aventyl*—Brand name no longer available
Protriptyline	20–60	5, 10	*Vivactil*—5, 10
Amoxapine	150–600	25, 50, 100, 150	*Ascendin*—Brand name no longer available
Trazodone	150–600	50, 100, 150	*Desyrel*—Brand name no longer available
Amitriptyline	100–300	10, 25, 50, 75, 100, 150	*Elavil*—Brand name no longer available *Limbitrol*—12.5 or 25 of amitriptyline with 5 or 10 of chlordiazepoxide; brand name no longer available *Triavil*—10, 25, or 50 of amitriptyline with perphenazine; brand name no longer available

Table App 3.2 RECOMMENDED TAPERING PROGRAMS FOR TRICYCLIC OR HETEROCYCLIC ANTIDEPRESSANTS

Find the dose of your antidepressant in the table and review the series of suggested dosage reductions to taper off the drug. The suggested reductions may need to be adjusted following the guidelines of the 5-Step Antidepressant Tapering Program, particularly if you have moderate to severe withdrawal reactions. All doses are in milligrams/day. Note: See Chapter 12 for guidelines on adjusting the dosage reductions for children and adolescents.

			600
300	150	60	450
200	100	40	300
100	50	20	150
50	25	10	75
0	0	0	0
Imipramine (Tofranil, Tofranil PM) Amitriptyline (Elavil, Limbitrol, Triavil) Desipramine (Norpramin) Trimipramine (Surmontil) Clomipramine (Anafranil) Doxepin (Sinequan) Maprotiline (Ludiomil)	Nortriptyline (Pamelor, Aventyl)	Protriptyline (Vivactil)	Amoxampine (Ascendin) Trazodone (Desyrel)

Tricyclic antidepressants boost serotonin and noradrenalin to varying degrees along with a number of other brain chemicals.[6] As a result, the withdrawal symptoms seen with tricyclics overlap considerably with those seen with today's popular antidepressants.[7] The psychiatric withdrawal symptoms of tricyclic antidepressants can mimic anxiety, depression, and mania, like today's antidepressants.[8] The same range of medical symptoms of withdrawal are possible, but with tricyclic antidepressants nausea, vomiting, and diarrhea, as well as flu-like symptoms are more common while dizziness, imbalance, and sensory abnormalities (burning, tingling, electric shock–like sensations, ringing in the ears, and visual abnormalities) are less common.[9] Stopping tricyclic antidepressants abruptly may also cause cardiac arrythmias, although this is unlikely when the drugs are tapered carefully.[10]

Table App. 3.2 provides recommended tapering programs for the tricyclic antidepressants. Working with your doctor to determine the recommended tapering program for you, find the dose of your antidepressant in the table and review the series of suggested dosage reductions to taper off the drug. These dosage reductions may need to be adjusted following the guidelines of the 5-Step Antidepressant Tapering Program, particularly if you have moderate to severe withdrawal reactions. If you are tapering a tricyclic or heterocyclic antidepressant, be sure to read this entire book before starting your taper to know the exceptions to the rules when tapering antidepressants and to have a full understanding of how the 5-Step Antidepressant Tapering Program works.

Appendix 4

Tapering Monoamine Oxidase Inhibitor Antidepressants

Monoamine oxidase inhibitor antidepressants, abbreviated MAOIs, are more stimulating than most of today's popular antidepressants. MAOIs boost the brain chemicals serotonin, noradrenalin, and dopamine by a different mechanism than today's popular antidepressants.[1] Their use is limited by severe toxic, potentially fatal, reactions to a variety of foods that cannot be eaten while on the drugs.[2] MAOIs also cause adverse reactions with a number of other drugs including over-the-counter medications. Because of the severe restrictions and risks, MAOIs tend to be antidepressants of last resort, used for patients who do not respond to less stimulating antidepressants. Since the October 2004 update, the FDA's warnings that people may become suicidal on antidepressants also apply to MAOIs.

Three MAOIs are currently on the market: tranylcypromine (whose brand name is Parnate), phenelzine (whose brand name is Nardil), and isocarboxazid (whose brand name is Marplan). MAOIs have amphetamine-like effects. In fact, after Parnate is ingested, it is converted by the liver into amphetamine.[3] As a result, if stopped abruptly, MAOIs can cause severe amphetamine-like withdrawal reactions, including delusions, hallucinations, agitation, and cognitive impairment that can be life threatening and require hospitalization.[4] While severe withdrawal reactions can occur with today's popular antidepressants, they are more common with MAOIs.[5] As a result, MAOIs have to be tapered extremely carefully under the supervision of a doctor with specialized expertise in prescribing these drugs. For this reason, I have not provided recommended tapering programs for patients on MAOIs. MAOIs should not be tapered by family doctors or even by psychiatrists who lack the specific expertise.

NOTES

In academic and professional journals, the chemical rather than the commercial names for drugs are typically used. For example, Prozac is referred to as fluoxetine. When these journals are quoted in the text, for readability, the well-recognized commercial names of the drugs have been substituted for their chemical names.

Preface

1. http://www.fda.gov/cder/drug/antidepressants/AntidepressantsPHA.htm.
2. C. Johnson, "Suicide warning ordered on drugs: antidepressant risk seen in youth," *Boston Globe*, October 16, 2004, p. A1; E. Shogren, "FDA orders depression drug warning; antidepressant labels will have to carry a prominent alert about the risk of suicidal thought and behavior in children and teens," *Los Angeles Times*, October 16, 2004, p. A8; G. Harris, "FDA toughens warning on antidepressant drugs," *The New York Times*, October 16, 2004, p. A9.
3. G. Harris, "F.D.A. links drugs to being suicidal," *The New York Times*, September 14, 2004, p. A1.
4. S. Vedantam, "FDA confirms antidepressants raise children's suicide risk," *The Washington Post*, September 14, 2004, p. A01.
5. Johnson, "Suicide warning ordered on drugs: antidepressant risk seen in youth." Note that Cymbalta is the newest of these antidepressants and was not yet on the market when the FDA issued its March 4, 2004 warning. Accordingly, Cymbalta was not one of the drugs as to which the FDA requested that a warning statement be used. However, Cymbalta is an SNRI-type antidepressant, in the same class as Effexor and Serzone, and when Eli Lilly launched Cymbalta in the summer of 2004, it incorporated the language of the FDA's March warning in its official information on Cymbalta. Cymbalta was included in the FDA's updated October 15, 2004 warning. In addition, the older tricyclic and monamine oxidase inhibitor antidepressants were added to the list of drugs covered by the warning at the time of the October 15 update. The October 2004 update added a black box warning on children and adoles-

cents and, at the same time, retained much of the language of the March 2004 warning on adults and children.

6. http://medicines.mhra.gove.uk/ourwork/monitorsafequalmed/safetymessages/ ssrioverview_101203.htm; S. Boseley, "Drugs for depressed children banned," *The Guardian*, December 10, 2003.

7. W. Kondro and B. Sibbald, "Drug company experts advised staff to withhold data about SSRI use in children," *Canadian Medical Association Journal* 2004;170(5):783.

8. SmithKlineBeecham [now GlaxoSmithKline], Central Medical Affairs team (CMAt), "Confidential, For Internal-Use Only Report: Paxil Adolescent Depression: position piece on the phase III clinical studies," October 1998.

9. Editorial, "Depressing research," *Lancet* 2004;363(9418):1335.

10. M. Keller et al., "Efficacy of paroxetine [Paxil] in the treatment of adolescent major depression: a randomized clinical trial," *Journal of the American Academy of Child and Adolescent Psychiatry* 2001;40(7):762–72.

11. Psychiatrists like Keller are not strangers to this controversy. Keller and a group of co-authors published an article on chronic, long-term use of antidepressants in patients in the May 18, 2000 issue of the *New England Journal of Medicine* [M. Keller et al., "A comparison of nefazodone (Serzone), the cognitive behavioral-analysis system of psychotherapy, and their combination for the treatment of chronic depression," *New England Journal of Medicine* 2000;342(20):1462–70]. In an accompanying editorial entitled "Is Academic Medicine for Sale?" the *New England Journal of Medicine* cited Keller and his co-authors as a "striking example" of the "ubiquitous" ties between prominent academic psychiatrists and the pharmaceutical industry [M. Angell, "Is academic medicine for sale?" Editorial, *New England Journal of Medicine* 2000;342:1516–18]. The *Journal* reported that Keller and his colleagues worked for so many pharmaceutical companies that there was not room to print all of them in the *Journal*, as they normally would. Instead they had to post them on their website. The editorial criticized the "cozy relations" between the pharmaceutical companies and the seemingly independent psychiatrists and revealed that many of the academic papers are "ghostwritten" by the companies for the authors who agree to put their names on them. In a rare glimpse into the kind of money involved in these "cozy relations," the *Boston Globe* revealed that Keller made $842,000 in 1998, earning more than half in consulting fees from pharmaceutical companies whose drugs he "lauded" in medical journals and or conferences [D. Kong and A. Bass, "Case at Brown leads to review," *Boston Globe*, October 8, 1999, p. B1]. Earning such fees on an annual basis, psychiatrists like Keller can earn millions of dollars consulting to pharmaceutical companies.

12. C. Whittington, T. Kendall, P. Fonagy, D. Cottrell, A. Cotgrove, E. Boddington, "Selective serotonin reuptake inhibitors in childhood depression: systematic review of published versus unpublished data, *Lancet* 2004;363:1341–5.

13. Editorial, "Depressing research."

14. B. Meier, "A.M.A urges disclosure on drug trials," *The New York Times,* June 16, 2004.

15. J. Jureidini and A. Tonkin, "Paroxetine [Paxil] in major depression," *Journal of the American Academy of Child and Adolescent Psychiatry* 2003;42(2): 514–5; M. Freudenheim, "Behavior drugs lead in sales for children," *The New York Times* May 17, 2004.

16. GlaxoSmithKline, "Dear Doctor" Letter, June 10, 2003, sent to doctors in the United Kingdom.

17. G. Harris, "New York State official sues drug maker over test data: Glaxo challenged in the use of Paxil for children," *The New York Times,* June 3, 2004, p. A1; B. Martinez, "Spitzer charges Glaxo concealed Paxil data," *Wall Street Journal,* June 3, 2004, p. B1.

18. B. Tansey, "Glaxo settles fraud suit: drug firm to post results of trials on its web site," *San Francisco Chronicle,* August 27, 2004.

19. Kong and Bass, "Case at Brown leads to review." Jureidini and Tonkin, "Paroxetine [Paxil] in major depression."

20. Angell, "Is academic medicine for sale?"; S. Brownlee, "Doctors without borders: why you can't trust medical journals anymore," *The Washington Monthly,* April 2004, pp. 38–43.

21. D. Healy, *Let Them Eat Prozac* (Toronto: James Lorimer, 2003).

22. Tansey, "Glaxo settles fraud suit."

23. R. Waters, "Drug report barred by FDA: scientist links antidepressants to suicide in kids," *San Francisco Chronicle,* February 1, 2004, p. A1; G. Harris, "Expert kept from speaking at antidepressant hearing," *The New York Times,* April 16, 2004, p. A16; E. Shogren, "FDA sat on report linking suicide, drugs," *Los Angeles Times,* April 6, 2004, p. A-13.

24. Harris, "F.D.A. links drugs to being suicidal."

25. R. Waters, "FDA was urged to limit kids' antidepressants: advice citing the risk of suicide rejected," *San Francisco Chronicle,* April 16, 2004, p. A1.

26. M. Kranish, "FDA counsel's rise embodies US shift," *Boston Globe,* December 22, 2002, p. A1; J. Glenmullen, *Prozac Backlash: Overcoming the Dangers of Prozac, Zoloft, Paxil, and Other Antidepressants with Safe, Effective Alternatives* (New York: Simon & Schuster, 2000), pp. 159–65.

27. Shogren, "FDA sat on report linking suicide, drugs."

28. Brownlee, "Doctors without borders."

29. M.J. Grinfeld, "Protecting Prozac," *California Lawyer,* December 1998, pp. 36–40, 79.

30. D. Kong, "Doctors fault service access: mental health care is concern," *Boston Globe,* October 16, 1997.

31. E. Shogren, "FDA probes downsides of antidepressants," *Los Angeles Times,* March 21, 2004, p. A15.

32. http://www.fda.gov/ohrms/dockets/ac/04/transcripts; 4006T1.htm.

33. Glenmullen, *Prozac Backlash.*
34. J.F. Rosenbaum, M. Fava, S.L. Hoog, R.C. Ascroft, W.B. Krebs, "Selective serotonin reuptake inhibitor discontinuation [withdrawal] syndrome: a randomized clinical trial," *Biological Psychiatry* 1998;44(2):77–87; M. Fava, R. Mulroy, J. Alpert, A.A. Nierenberg, J.F. Rosenbaum, "Emergence of adverse events following discontinuation [withdrawal] of treatment with extended-release venlafaxine [Effexor]," *American Journal of Psychiatry* 1997; 154(12):1760–2.

Chapter 1. Antidepressant Withdrawal and Dependence

1. M. Fava, R. Mulroy, J. Alpert, A.A. Nierenberg, J.F. Rosenbaum, "Emergence of adverse events following discontinuation [withdrawal] of treatment with extended-release venlafaxine [Effexor]," *American Journal of Psychiatry* 1997;154(12):1760–2.
2. P.M. Haddad, "Antidepressant discontinuation [withdrawal] syndromes," *Drug Safety* 2001;24(3):183–97; M. Lejoyeux, J. Ades, I. Mourad, J. Solomon, S. Dilsaver, "Antidepressant withdrawal syndrome: recognition, prevention and management," *CNS Drugs* 1996;4:278–92; GlaxoSmithKline, Official product information (product insert) for Deroxat [the Swiss name for Paxil], January 9, 1997, English translation.
3. J.G. Hardman and L.E. Limbird, Eds., *Goodman & Gilman's The Pharmacological Basis of Therapeutics,* 10th Edition (New York: McGraw-Hill, 2001), p. 626. This is the standard textbook of pharmacology, covering all of medicine not just psychiatry. The definition of dependence is that the patient "requires continued administration of the drug to maintain normal function." The authoritative textbook specifically states that people can become dependent on prescription medications: "Patients who take medicine for appropriate medical indications and in correct dose may still show tolerance, physical dependence, and withdrawal symptoms if the drug is stopped abruptly rather than gradually." According to this standard medical definition, antidepressants can clearly cause dependence. But, pharmaceutical companies sometimes try to deny that antidepressants cause dependence by hiding behind another term, "substance dependence," defined in the American Psychiatric Association's *Diagnostic and Statistical Manual* as a syndrome of escalating drug use that impairs social and occupational performance. But "substance dependence" as so defined is not the same thing as dependence and pharmaceutical companies are playing semantic gamesmanship when trying to hide behind this term. See: American Psychiatric Association, *Diagnostic and Statistical Manual of Mental Disorders,* 4th Ed. (Washington, DC: American Psychiatric Association, 1994), pp. 176–81.
4. K. Demyttenaere and P. Haddad, "Compliance with antidepressant therapy

and antidepressant discontinuation [withdrawal] symptoms," *Acta Psychiatrica Scandinavica* 2000;101(suppl 403):50–6; K. Demyttenaere, E. Van Ganse, J. Gregoire, E. Gaens, P. Mesters, "Compliance in depressed patients treated with fluoxetine [Prozac] or amitriptyline. Belgian Compliance Study Group," *International Clinical Psychopharmacology* 1998;13(1):11–17; K. Demyttenaere, "Compliance during treatment with antidepressants," *Journal of Affective Disorders* 1997;43:27–39.

5. E. Shogren, "FDA probes downsides of antidepressants," *Los Angeles Times,* March 21, 2004, p. A15.

6. C. Thompson, "Discontinuation [Withdrawal] of antidepressant therapy: emerging complications and their relevance," *Journal of Clinical Psychiatry* 1998;59(10):541–8.

7. S. Nuss, C.R. Kincaid, "Serotonin discontinuation [withdrawal] syndrome: does it really exist?" *West Virginia Medical Journal* 2000;96(2):405–7; Haddad, "Antidepressant discontinuation [withdrawal] syndromes"; D.W. Black, R. Wesner, J. Gabel, "The abrupt discontinuation [withdrawal] of fluvoxamine [Luvox] in patients with panic disorder," *Journal of Clinical Psychiatry* 1993;54(4):146–9; Thompson, "Discontinuation [Withdrawal] of antidepressant therapy; Lejoyeux et al., "Antidepressant withdrawal syndrome: recognition, prevention and management."

8. A.H. Young, A. Currie, "Physicians' knowledge of antidepressant withdrawal effects: a survey," *Journal of Clinical Psychiatry* 1997;58(suppl 7):28–30; M. J. Grinfeld, "Protecting Prozac," *California Lawyer,* December 1998, pp. 36–40, 79. See also E.J. Pollock, "Managed care's focus on psychiatric drugs alarms many doctors," *Wall Street Journal,* December 1, 1995, p. 1.

9. J.F. Rosenbaum, M. Fava, S.L. Hoog, R.C. Ascroft, W.B. Krebs, "Selective serotonin reuptake inhibitor discontinuation [withdrawal] syndrome: a randomized clinical trial," *Biological Psychiatry* 1998;44(2):77–87.

10. J.S. Price, P.C. Waller, S.M. Wood, A.V. MacKay, "A comparison of the post-marketing safety of four selective serotonin re-uptake inhibitors including the investigation of symptoms occurring on withdrawal," *British Journal of Clinical Pharmacology* 1996;42(6):757–63.

11. *Australian Adverse Drug Reactions Bulletin,* "SSRIs and withdrawal syndrome," 1996;15(1); R. M. Lane, "Withdrawal symptoms after discontinuation of selective serotonin reuptake inhibitors (SSRIs)," *Journal of Serotonin Research,* 1996;3:75–83; P. Haddad, "Newer antidepressants and the discontinuation [withdrawal] syndrome," *Journal of Clinical Psychiatry* 1997;58 (suppl 7):17–21, discussion 22; Rosenbaum et al., "Selective serotonin reuptake inhibitor discontinuation [withdrawal] syndrome"; F.J. Mackay, N.R. Dunn, L.V. Wilton, G.L. Pearce, S.N. Freemantle, R.D. Mann, "A Comparison of fluvoxamine [Luvox], fluoxetine [Prozac], sertraline [Zoloft], and paroxetine [Paxil] examined by observational cohort studies," *Pharmacoepidemiology and Drug Safety* 1997;6:235–46.

12. Black et al., "The abrupt discontinuation [withdrawal] of fluvoxamine [Luvox] in patients with panic disorder."

13. F. Bogetto, S. Bellino, R.B. Revello, L. Patria, "Discontinuation [withdrawal] syndrome in dysthymic patients treated with selective serotonin reuptake inhibitors: a clinical investigation," *CNS Drugs* 2002;16(4):273–83; M. Lejoyeux, J. Ades, "Antidepressant discontinuation [withdrawal]: a review of the literature," *Journal of Clinical Psychiatry* 1997;58(7):11–15, discussion 16; Rosenbaum et al., "Selective serotonin reuptake inhibitor discontinuation [withdrawal] syndrome"; A.F. Schatzberg, "Antidepressant discontinuation [withdrawal] syndrome: an update on serotonin reuptake inhibitors," *Journal of Clinical Psychiatry* 1997;58(7):3–4; J. Zajecka, K.A. Tracy, S. Mitchell, "Discontinuation [Withdrawal] symptoms after treatment with serotonin reuptake inhibitors: a literature review," *Journal of Clinical Psychiatry* 1997;58(7): 291–7.

14. http://www.fda.gov/cder/drug/antidepressants/AntidepressanstPHA.htm.

15. M. Bloch, S.V. Stager, A.R. Braun, D.R. Rubinow, "Severe psychiatric symptoms associated with paroxetine [Paxil] withdrawal," *Lancet* 1995;346(8966): 57; F. Benazzi, "Sertraline [Zoloft] discontinuation [withdrawal] syndrome presenting with severe depression and compulsions," *Biological Psychiatry* 1998;43(12):929–30; L.F. Koopowitz, M. Berk, "Paroxetine [Paxil]-induced withdrawal effects," *Human Psychopharmacology* 1995;10:147–8.

16. J. Glenmullen, *Prozac Backlash: Overcoming the Dangers of Prozac, Zoloft, Paxil, and Other Antidepressants with Safe, Effective Alternatives* (New York: Simon & Schuster, 2000).

17. P. Haddad, "The SSRI discontinuation [withdrawal] syndrome," *Journal of Psychopharmacology* 1998;12(3):305–13.

18. J. Winkelman, C. Dorsey, S. Cunningham et al., "Fluoxetine [Prozac] produces persistent rapid eye movements in non-REM sleep," *Sleep Research* 1992;21:78; R. Armitage, M. Trivedi, A.J. Rush, "Fluoxetine [Prozac] and oculomotor activity during sleep in depressed patients," *Neuropsychopharmacology* 1995;12(2):159–65; C.H. Schneck, M.W. Mahowald, S.W. Kim et al. "Prominent eye movements during NREM sleep and REM sleep behavior disorder associated with fluoxetine [Prozac] treatment of depression and obsessive-compulsive disorder," *Sleep* 1992;15(3):226–35.

19. R.J. Baldessarini, "Risks and implications of interrupting maintenance psychotropic drug therapy," *Psychotherapy and Psychosomatics* 1995;63(3–4): 137–41.

20. *Drug and Therapeutics Bulletin* [No authors listed], "Withdrawing patients from antidepressants," 1999;37(7):49–52.

21. B. Sadock and V. Sadock, *Kaplan and Sadock's Synopsis of Psychiatry,* 9th Ed. (Philadelphia: Lippincott Williams & Wilkins, 2003), p. 569.

22. Haddad, "The SSRI discontinuation [withdrawal] syndrome."

23. A.F. Schatzberg, P. Haddad, E.M. Kaplan, M. Lejoyeux, J.F. Rosenbaum, A.H.

Young, J. Zajecka, "Possible biological mechanisms of the serotonin reuptake inhibitor discontinuation [withdrawal] syndrome. Discontinuation Consensus Panel," *Journal of Clinical Psychiatry* 1997;58(7):23–7.

24. Haddad, "Antidepressant discontinuation [withdrawal] syndromes."

25. *Physician's Desk Reference (PDR)*, (Montvale, NJ: Thomson PDR, 2004), pp. 1583–94. GlaxoSmithKline added the caution in December 2001.

26. Glenmullen, *Prozac Backlash*, pp. 64–104.

27. J.F. Rosenbaum et al. "Selective serotonin reuptake inhibitor discontinuation [withdrawal] syndrome"; Fava et al., "Emergence of adverse events following discontinuation [withdrawal] of treatment with extended-release venlafaxine [Effexor]."

28. N.J. Coupland, C.J. Bell, J.P. Potokar, "Serotonin reuptake inhibitor withdrawal," *Journal of Clinical Psychopharmacology* 1996;16(5):356–62.

29. C. Debattista and A.F. Schatzberg, "Physical symptoms associated with paroxetine [Paxil] withdrawal," *American Journal of Psychiatry* 1995;152(8): 1235–6.

30. A. Farah and T.E. Lauer, "Possible venlafaxine [Effexor] withdrawal syndrome," *American Journal of Psychiatry* 1996;153(4):576.

31. J.F. Rosenbaum and J. Zajecka, "Clinical management of antidepressant discontinuation [withdrawal]," *Journal of Clinical Psychiatry* 1997;58(suppl 7):37–40.

32. L. Frost and S. Lal, "Shock-like sensations after discontinuation of selective serotonin reuptake inhibitors," *American Journal of Psychiatry* 1995 May; 152(5):810.

33. R.S. Diler, L. Tamam, A. Avci, "Withdrawal symptoms associated with paroxetine [Paxil] discontinuation in a nine-year-old boy," *Journal of Clinical Psychopharmacology* 2000;20(5):586–7.

34. M.L. Dahl, E. Olhager, J. Ahlner, "Paroxetine [Paxil] withdrawal syndrome in a neonate," *British Journal of Psychiatry* 1997;171:391–2.

35. L.S. Kent and J.D. Laidlaw, "Suspected congenital sertraline [Zoloft] dependence," *British Journal of Psychiatry* 1995;167(3):412–3.

36. Haddad, "Antidepressant discontinuation [withdrawal] syndromes."

37. G. Cowley, "The Promise of Prozac," cover story, *Newsweek,* March 26, 1990, p. 38.

38. A.F. Schatzberg, P. Haddad, E.M. Kaplan, M. Lejoyeux, J.F. Rosenbaum, A.H. Young, J. Zajecka, "Serotonin reuptake inhibitor discontinuation [withdrawal] syndrome: hypothetical definition," *Journal of Clinical Psychiatry* 1997;58(suppl 7):5–10.

39. *PDR,* 2004, pp. 3413–18; *PDR,* 2000, pp. 849–53. Noradrenalin is also called norepinephrine.

40. S. Todd, "Bristol's Serzone pulled off market—Antidepressant is linked to liver injury," *Star-Ledger* (Newark, NJ), May 20, 2004.

41. *PDR,* 2004, pp. 2389–92.

42. Ibid. pp. 1658–61.

43. Fava et al., "Emergence of adverse events following discontinuation [withdrawal] of treatment with extended-release venlafaxine [Effexor]."

44. J.F. Rosenbaum et al., "Selective serotonin reuptake inhibitor discontinuation [withdrawal] syndrome."

45. S.C. Dilsaver, J.F. Greden, "Antidepressant withdrawal phenomena," *Biological Psychiatry* 1984;19(2):237–56; S.C. Dilsaver, "Withdrawal phenomena associated with antidepressant and antipsychotic agents," *Drug Safety* 1994;10(2):103–14; J.F. Rosenbaum et al., "Selective serotonin reuptake inhibitor discontinuation [withdrawal] syndrome."

46. R. Hales and S. Yudofsky, *Essentials of Clinical Psychiatry,* 2nd Ed. (Washington, DC: American Psychiatric Publishing, 2000), p. 810.

47. C. Sherman, "Long-term side effects surface with SSRIs," *Clinical Psychiatry News,* May 1998, pp. 1, 8.

48. Studies in which patients on SSRIs are directly asked about sexual dysfunction have found rates as high as 60 percent or more of patients. One of the earliest systematic studies of 60 patients found this high rate. See W.M. Patterson, "Fluoxetine [Prozac]-induced sexual dysfunction," *Journal of Clinical Psychiatry* 1993;54:71. Large-scale studies include that of Modell, who found rates of sexual side effects of 73 percent for Prozac, 67 percent for Zoloft, and 86 percent for Paxil. See J. G. Modell, C. R. Katholi, J.D. Modell, and R.L. DePalma, "Comparative sexual side effects of bupropion [Wellbutrin], fluoxetine [Prozac], paroxetine [Paxil], and sertraline [Zoloft]," *Clinical Pharmacology and Therapeutics* 1997;61:476–87. The most comprehensive study was that of the Montejo-González group, who found an overall rate of 58 percent of patients on Prozac, Zoloft, Paxil, or Luvox reporting sexual side effects. See A.L. Montejo-González, G. Llorca, J.A. Izquierdo, A. Ledesma, M. Bousono, A. Calcedo, J.L. Carrasco, J. Ciudad, E. Daniel, J. De la Gandra, J. Derecho, M. Franco, M.J. Gomez, J. A. Macias, T. Martin, V. Perez, J.M. Sanchez, S. Sanchez, and E. Vicens, "SSRI-induced sexual dysfunction: fluoxetine [Prozac], paroxetine [Paxil], sertraline [Zoloft], and fluvoxamine [Luvox] in a prospective, multicenter, and descriptive clinical study of 344 patients," *Journal of Sex and Marital Therapy,* 1997;(23):176–94.

49. Glenmullen, *Prozac Backlash,* pp. 39–43.

50. M. Fava, S.M. Rappe, J.A. Pava, A.A. Nierenbergh, J.E. Alpert, and J.F. Rosenbaum, "Relapse in patients on long-term fluoxetine [Prozac] treatment: response to increased fluoxetine dose," *Journal of Clinical Psychiatry* 1995;56:52–55.

51. S. Fried, "Addicted to anti-depressants? The controversy over a pill millions of us are taking," *Glamour,* April 2003, pp. 178–80, 262.

Chapter 2. Resolving the Controversy over "Addiction" to Antidepressants

1. M. Fava, S.M. Rappe, J.A. Pava, A.A. Nierenbergh, J.E. Alpert, and J.F. Rosenbaum, "Relapse in patients on long-term fluoxetine [Prozac] treatment: response to increased fluoxetine [Prozac] dose," *Journal of Clinical Psychiatry* 1995;56:52–55.

2. F. Gardner, "Prozac 'Abuse,' " *Anderson Valley Advertiser* (Boonville, CA), February 23, 1994, p. 5.

3. D. Amsden, "Generation Rx: Pop, Snort, Parachute," *New York*, October 4, 2004.

4. P. Kramer, *Listening to Prozac* (New York: Viking, 1993), p. 244.

5. *Oxford English Dictionary*, 2nd Ed. (Oxford: Clarendon Press, 1989), p. 143.

6. J.F. Rosenbaum, M. Fava, S.L. Hoog, R.C. Ascroft, W.B. Krebs, "Selective serotonin reuptake inhibitor discontinuation [withdrawal] syndrome: a randomized clinical trial," *Biological Psychiatry* 1998;44(2):77–87; D.W. Black, R. Wesner, J. Gabel, "The abrupt discontinuation [withdrawal] of fluvoxamine [Luvox] in patients with panic disorder," *Journal of Clinical Psychiatry* 1993;54(4):146–9; M. Fava, R. Mulroy, J. Alpert, A.A. Nierenberg, J.F. Rosenbaum, "Emergence of adverse events following discontinuation [withdrawal] of treatment with extended-release venlafaxine [Effexor]," *American Journal of Psychiatry* 1997;154(12):1760–2.

7. *Journal of Clinical Psychiatry*, 1997;58(suppl 7): see inside cover for statement of Lilly sponsorship.

8. A.F. Schatzberg, P. Haddad, E.M. Kaplan, M. Lejoyeux, J.F. Rosenbaum, A.H. Young, and J. Zajecka, "Serotonin reuptake inhibitor discontinuation [withdrawal] syndrome: hypothetical definition," *Journal of Clinical Psychiatry* 1997;58(suppl 7):5–10.

9. A.F. Schatzberg, "Introduction: antidepressant discontinuation [withdrawal] syndrome: an update on serotonin reuptake inhibitors," *Journal of Clinical Psychiatry* 1997;58(suppl 7):3–4; Schatzberg et al., "Serotonin reuptake inhibitor discontinuation [withdrawal] syndrome;" M. Lejoyeux and J. Adés, "Antidepressant discontinuation [withdrawal]: a review of the literature," *Journal of Clinical Psychiatry* 1997;58(suppl 7):11–16; P. Haddad, "Newer antidepressants and the discontinuation [withdrawal] syndrome," *Journal of Clinical Psychiatry* 1997;58(suppl 7):17–22; A.F. Schatzberg, P. Haddad, E.M. Kaplan, M. Lejoyeux, J.F. Rosenbaum, A.H. Young, J. Zajecka, "Possible biological mechanisms of the serotonin reuptake inhibitor discontinuation [withdrawal] syndrome," *Journal of Clinical Psychiatry* 1997;58(suppl 7):23–27; A.H. Young and A. Currie, "Physicians' knowledge of antidepressant withdrawal effects: a survey," *Journal of Clinical Psychiatry* 1997;58(suppl 7):28–30; E.M. Kaplan, "Antidepressant noncompliance as a factor in the discontinuation [withdrawal] syndrome, *Journal of Clinical Psychiatry* 1997;

58(suppl 7):31–36; J. F. Rosenbaum and J. Zajecka, "Clinical management of antidepressant discontinuation [withdrawal]," *Journal of Clinical Psychiatry* 1997;58(suppl 7):37–40.

10. *Physician's Desk Reference (PDR)*, (Montvale, NJ: Thomson PDR, 2004), pp. 1583–94.

11. Ibid., pp. 3413–24.

12. *Panorama*, "The Secrets of Seroxat [Paxil]," The British Broadcasting Company (BBC), October 13, 2002; *Panorama*, "Seroxat [Paxil]: Emails from the Edge," BBC, May 11, 2003. Note: the British name for Paxil is Seroxat.

13. C. Medawar, A. Herxheimer, A. Bell, S. Jofre, "Paroxetine [Paxil], *Panorama* and user reporting of ADRs: consumer intelligence matters in clinical practice and post-marketing drug surveillance," *International Journal of Risk & Safety in Medicine*, 2002;15:161–69.

14. D. Healy, *The Antidepressant Era* (Cambridge: Harvard University Press, 1997), p. 367.

15. C. Medawar and A. Hardon, *Medicines Out of Control?* (The Netherlands: Askant Academic Publishers, 2004).

16. GlaxoSmithKline, " 'Seroxat' [Paxil] (paroxetine) Tablets Patient Information Leaflet," July 2001.

17. GlaxoSmithKline, "Dear Doctor" Letter, June 18, 2003, sent to doctors in the United Kingdom.

18. GlaxoSmithKline, "Dear Doctor" Letter, May 8, 2003, sent to doctors in the United Kingdom.

19. R. Woodman, "UK replaces team reviewing safety of SSRIs," Reuters Health, London, March 26, 2003.

20. P.M. Haddad and M. Qureshi, "Misdiagnosis of antidepressant discontinuation [withdrawal] symptoms," *Acta Psychiatrica Scandinavica* 2000;102(6): 466–7; P. Tyrer, "Invited commentary," *Acta Psychiatrica Scandinavica* 2000; 102(6):467–8; *Drug and Therapeutics Bulletin* [No authors listed], "Withdrawing patients from antidepressants," 1999;37(7):49–52.

21. J.G. Hardman and L.E. Limbird, Eds., *Goodman & Gilman's The Pharmacological Basis of Therapeutics*, 10th Edition (New York: McGraw-Hill, 2001), p. 626. See note 3 in Chapter 1 (p. 216).

Chapter 3. The Withdrawal Spectrum

1. F. Benazzi, "SSRI discontinuation [withdrawal] syndrome related to fluvoxamine [Luvox]," *Journal of Psychiatry and Neuroscience* 1998;23(2):94; M. Bloch, S.V. Stager, A.R. Braun, D.R. Rubinow, "Severe psychiatric symptoms associated with paroxetine [Paxil] withdrawal," *Lancet* 1995;346(8966):571.

2. F. Bogetto, S. Bellino, R.B. Revello, L. Patria, "Discontinuation [Withdrawal] syndrome in dysthymic patients treated with selective serotonin reuptake inhibitors: a clinical investigation," *CNS Drugs* 2002;16(4):273–83; P. Haddad,

"The SSRI discontinuation [withdrawal] syndrome," *Journal of Psychopharmacology* 1998;12(3):305–13; P.M. Haddad, "Antidepressant discontinuation [withdrawal] syndromes," *Drug Safety* 2001;24(3):183–97; P. Haddad, "Newer antidepressants and the discontinuation [withdrawal] syndrome," *Journal of Clinical Psychiatry* 1997;58(suppl 7):17–21, discussion 22; *Australian Adverse Drug Reactions Bulletin*, "SSRIs and withdrawal syndrome," 1996;15(1).

3. A.F. Schatzberg, P. Haddad, E.M. Kaplan, M. Lejoyeux, J.F. Rosenbaum, A.H. Young, J. Zajecka, "Serotonin reuptake inhibitor discontinuation [withdrawal] syndrome: a hypothetical definition. Discontinuation Consensus panel," *Journal of Clinical Psychiatry* 1997;58(suppl 7):5–10; R.A. Dominguez and P.J. Goodnick, "Adverse events after the abrupt discontinuation [withdrawal] of paroxetine [Paxil]," *Pharmacotherapy* 1995;15(6):778–80; M.C.Miller, "Symptoms that start when an antidepressant stops," *Harvard Mental Health Letter* 2001;17(8):7–8.

4. A.K. Louie, R.A. Lannon, L.J. Ajari, "Withdrawal reaction after sertraline [Zoloft] discontinuation [withdrawal]," *American Journal of Psychiatry* 1994;151(3):450–1; F.L. Leiter, A.A. Nierenberg, K.M. Sanders, T.A. Stern, "Discontinuation [withdrawal] reactions following sertraline [Zoloft]," *Biological Psychiatry* 1995;38(10):694–5; C. Debattista and A.F. Schatzberg, "Physical symptoms associated with paroxetine [Paxil] withdrawal," *American Journal of Psychiatry* 1995;152(8):1235–6; F. Benazzi, "Sertraline [Zoloft] discontinuation [withdrawal] syndrome presenting with severe depression and compulsions," *Biological Psychiatry* 1998;43(12):929–30; F. Bogetto et al., "Discontinuation [Withdrawal] syndrome in dysthymic patients treated with selective serotonin reuptake inhibitors."

5. D.K. Arya, "Withdrawal after discontinuation of paroxetine [Paxil]," *Australian and New Zealand Journal of Psychiatry* 1996;30(5):702.

6. R.E. Pyke, "Paroxetine [Paxil] withdrawal syndrome," *American Journal of Psychiatry* 1995;152(1):149–50; Dominguez and Goodnick, "Adverse events after the abrupt discontinuation [withdrawal] of paroxetine [Paxil]."

7. L.C. Barr, W.K. Goodman, L.H. Price, "Physical symptoms associated with paroxetine [Paxil] discontinuation [withdrawal]," *American Journal of Psychiatry* 1994;151(2):289.

8. Dominguez and Goodnick, "Adverse events after the abrupt discontinuation [withdrawal] of paroxetine [Paxil]"; Schatzberg et al., "Serotonin reuptake inhibitor discontinuation [withdrawal] syndrome."

9. Schatzberg et al., "Serotonin reuptake inhibitor discontinuation [withdrawal] syndrome."

10. L.F. Koopowitz and M. Berk, "Paroxetine [Paxil]-induced withdrawal effects," *Human Psychopharmacology* 1995;10:147–8; Bloch et al., "Severe psychiatric symptoms associated with paroxetine [Paxil] withdrawal"; Benazzi, "Sertraline [Zoloft] discontinuation [withdrawal] syndrome presenting with severe depression and compulsions."

11. Bloch et al., "Severe psychiatric symptoms associated with paroxetine [Paxil] withdrawal."

12. Koopowitz and Berk, "Paroxetine [Paxil]-induced withdrawal effects."

13. GlaxoSmithKline, "Dear Doctor" letter, June 10, 2003, sent to doctors in the United Kingdom; A "frequent" side effect is officially defined as one that occurs in more than 1% of patients.

14. http://www.fda.gov/cder/drug/antidepressants/AntidepressantsPHA.htm.

15. J.S. Price, P.C. Waller, S.M. Wood, A.V. MacKay, "A comparison of the post-marketing safety of four selective serotonin re-uptake inhibitors including the investigation of symptoms occurring on withdrawal," *British Journal of Clinical Pharmacology* 1996;42(6):757–63; M. Lejoyeux and J. Ades, "Antidepressant discontinuation [withdrawal]: a review of the literature," *Journal of Clinical Psychiatry* 1997;58(suppl 7):11–5; discussion 16; A.L. Lazowick, G.M. Levin, "Potential withdrawal syndrome associated with SSRI discontinuation [withdrawal]," *Annals of Pharmacotherapy* 1995;29(12):1284–85; Benazzi, "Sertraline [Zoloft] discontinuation [withdrawal] syndrome presenting with severe depression and compulsions";43(12):929–30; C. Milliken and S.J. Cooper, "Withdrawal symptoms from Paroxetine [Paxil]," *Human Psychopharmacology* 1998;13:217–9; J.F. Rosenbaum, M. Fava, S.L. Hoog, R.C. Ascroft, W.B. Krebs, "Selective serotonin reuptake inhibitor discontinuation [withdrawal] syndrome: a randomized clinical trial," *Biological Psychiatry* 1998;44(2):77–87; D. Michelson, M. Fava, J. Amsterdam, J. Apter, P. Londborg, R. Tamura, R.G. Tepner, "Interruption of selective serotonin reuptake inhibitor treatment. Double-blind, placebo-controlled trial," *British Journal of Psychiatry* 2000;176:363–8; L.S. Kent, J.D. Laidlaw, "Suspected congenital sertraline [Zoloft] dependence," *British Journal of Psychiatry* 1995;167(3): 412–3.

16. D. Shoenberger, "Discontinuing [Withdrawing from] paroxetine [Paxil]: a personal account," *Psychotherapy and Psychosomatics* 2002;71(4):237–8.

17. Benazzi, "SSRI discontinuation [withdrawal] syndrome related to fluvoxamine" [Luvox]; Block et al., "Severe psychiatric symptoms associated with paroxetine [Paxil] withdrawal."

18. GlaxoSmithKline, "Dear Doctor" Letter, June 10, 2003; C. Medawar, A. Herxheimer, A. Bell, S. Jofre, "Paroxetine [Paxil], *Panorama*, and user reporting of ADRs: consumer intelligence matters in clinical practice and post-marketing drug surveillance," *International Journal of Risk & Safety in Medicine* 2002;15:161–69.

19. E. Szabadi, "Fluvoxamine [Luvox] withdrawal syndrome," *British Journal of Psychiatry* 1992;160:283–4.

20. A.K. Louie, R.A. Lannon, L.J. Ajari, "Withdrawal reaction after sertraline [Zoloft] discontinuation [withdrawal]," *American Journal of Psychiatry* 1994;151(3):450–1; L. Belloeuf, C. Le Jeunne, F.C. Hugues, "Paroxetine [Paxil] withdrawal syndrome," *Annales de Medicine Interne* (Paris) 2000;151

(suppl A)A52–3; D.K. Arya, "Withdrawal after discontinuation of paroxetine [Paxil]," *Australian and New Zealand Journal of Psychiatry* 1996;30(5):702.

21. D. Kasantikul, "Reversible delirium after discontinuation [withdrawal] of fluoxetine [Prozac]," *Journal of the Medical Association of Thailand* 1995; 78(1):53–4; G. Parker and J. Blennerhassett, "Withdrawal reactions associated with venlafaxine [Effexor]," *Australian and New Zealand Journal of Psychiatry* 1998;32(2):291–4.

22. Michelson et al., "Interruption of selective serotonin reuptake inhibitor treatment"; P. Landry and L. Roy, "Withdrawal hypomania associated with paroxetine [Paxil]," *Journal of Clinical Psychopharmacology* 1997;17(1):60–1.

23. Dominguez and Goodnick, "Adverse events after the abrupt discontinuation [withdrawal] of paroxetine [Paxil]"; K. Black, C. Shea, S. Dursun, S. Kutcher, "Selective serotonin re-uptake inhibitor discontinuation [withdrawal] syndrome: proposed diagnostic criteria," *Journal of Psychiatry and Neuroscience* 2000;25(3):255–61.

24. C.S. Berlin, "Fluoxetine [Prozac] withdrawal symptoms," *Journal of Clinical Psychiatry* 1996;57(2):93–4; D.W. Black, R. Wesner, J. Gabel, "The abrupt discontinuation [withdrawal] of fluvoxamine [Luvox] in patients with panic disorder," *Journal of Clinical Psychiatry* 1993;54(4):146–9; P.M. Haddad, S. Devarajan, S.M. Dursun, "Antidepressant discontinuation [withdrawal] symptoms presenting as 'stroke,'" *Journal of Psychopharmacology* 2001; 15(2):139–41.

25. Black et al., "The abrupt discontinuation [withdrawal] of fluvoxamine [Luvox] in patients with panic disorder"; Michelson et al., "Interruption of selective serotonin reuptake inhibitor treatment"; J.F. Rosenbaum, J. Zajecka, "Clinical management of antidepressant discontinuation [withdrawal]," *Journal of Clinical Psychiatry* 1997;58(suppl 7):37–40; Barr et al., "Physical symptoms associated with paroxetine [Paxil] discontinuation [withdrawal]."

26. Black et al., "Selective serotonin reuptake inhibitor discontinuation [withdrawal] syndrome: proposed diagnostic criteria"; S. Oehrberg, P.E. Christiansen, K. Behnke, A.L. Borup, B. Severin, J. Soegaard, H. Calberg, R. Judge, J.K. Ohrstrom, P.M. Manniche, "Paroxetine [Paxil] in the treatment of panic disorder. A randomised, double-blind, placebo-controlled study," *British Journal of Psychiatry* 1995;167(3):374–9; Haddad, "Antidepressant discontinuation [withdrawal] syndromes."

27. N.J. Coupland, C.J. Bell, J.P. Potokar, "Serotonin reuptake inhibitor withdrawal," *Journal of Clinical Psychopharmacology* 1996;16(5):356–62.

28. Berlin, "Fluoxetine [Prozac] withdrawal symptoms"; Coupland et al., "Serotonin reuptake inhibitor withdrawal"; A.F. Schatzberg, P. Haddad, E.M. Kaplan, M. Lejoyeux, J.F. Rosenbaum, A.H. Young, J. Zajecka, "Possible biological mechanisms of the serotonin reuptake inhibitor discontinuation [withdrawal] syndrome. Discontinuation Consensus Panel," *Journal of Clinical Psychiatry* 1997;58(suppl 7):23–7.

29. Schatzberg et al., "Possible biological mechanisms of the serotonin reuptake inhibitor discontinuation [withdrawal] syndrome"; Coupland et al., "Serotonin reuptake inhibitor withdrawal."

30. H.A. Rosenstock, "Sertraline [Zoloft] withdrawal in two brothers: a case report," *International Clinical Psychopharmacology* 1996;11(1):58–9; N.J. Keuthen, P. Cyr, J.A. Ricciardi, W.E. Minichiello, M.L. Buttolph, M.A. Jenike, "Medication withdrawal symptoms in obsessive-compulsive disorder patients treated with paroxetine [Paxil]," *Journal of Clinical Psychopharmacology* 1994;14(3):206–7; L. Frost and S. Lal, "Shock-like sensations after discontinuation [withdrawal] of selective serotonin reuptake inhibitors," *American Journal of Psychiatry* 1995;152(5):810; Lejoyeux and Ades, "Antidepressant discontinuation [withdrawal]: a review of the literature"; Koopowitz and Berk, "Paroxetine [Paxil]-induced withdrawal effects."

31. Koopowitz and Berk, "Paroxetine [Paxil]-induced withdrawal effects."

32. Pyke, "Paroxetine [Paxil] withdrawal syndrome"; A. Lazowick, "Potential withdrawal syndrome associated with SSRI discontinuation," *Annals of Pharmacotherapy* 1995;29:1284–85; Keuthen et al., "Medication withdrawal symptoms in obsessive-compulsive disorder patients treated with paroxetine [Paxil]."

33. Keuthen et al., "Medication withdrawal symptoms in obsessive-compulsive disorder patients treated with paroxetine [Paxil]"; T. Trenque, D. Piednoir, C. Frances, H. Millart, M.L. Germain, "Reports of withdrawal syndrome with the use of SSRIs: a case/non-case study in the French Pharmacovigilance database," *Pharmacoepidemiology and Drug Safety* 2002;11(4):281–3.

34. Haddad, "Antidepressant discontinuation [withdrawal] syndromes."

35. J. Glenmullen, *Prozac Backlash: Overcoming the Dangers of Prozac, Zoloft, Paxil, and Other Antidepressants with Safe, Effective Alternatives* (New York: Simon & Schuster, 2000), pp. 64–76; G. Mallya, K. White, C. Gunderson, "Is there a serotonergic withdrawal syndrome?" *Biological Psychiatry* 1993;33 (11–12):851–2; J.M. Ellison, "SSRI withdrawal buzz," *Journal of Clinical Psychiatry* 1994;55(12):544–5.

36. Rosenstock, "Sertraline [Zoloft] withdrawal in two brothers: a case report"; Frost and Lal, "Shock-like sensations after discontinuation [withdrawal] of selective serotonin reuptake inhibitors"; Dominguez and Goodnick, "Adverse events after the abrupt discontinuation [withdrawal] of paroxetine [Paxil]"; R.M. Lane, "Withdrawal symptoms after discontinuation [withdrawal] of selective serotonin reuptake inhibitors (SSRIs)," *Journal of Serotonin Research,* 1996;3:75–83; Coupland et al., "Serotonin reuptake inhibitor withdrawal."

37. R.R. Reeves and H.B. Pinkofsky, "Lhermitte's sign in paroxetine [Paxil] withdrawal," *Journal of Clinical Psychopharmacology* 1996;16(5):411–2.

38. Barr et al., "Physical symptoms associated with paroxetine [Paxil] discontinuation [withdrawal]."

39. Black et al., "The abrupt discontinuation [withdrawal] of fluvoxamine [Luvox] in patients with panic disorder."

40. *Australian Adverse Drug Reactions Bulletin*, "SSRIs and withdrawal syndrome"; Rosenbaum et al., "Selective serotonin reuptake inhibitor discontinuation [withdrawal] syndrome."

41. *Physician's Desk Reference (PDR)*, (Montvale, NJ: Thomson PDR, 2004), pp. 2389–92.

42. F. Benazzi, "Mirtazapine [Remeron] withdrawal symptoms," *Canadian Journal of Psychiatry* 1998;43(4):525; J. Klesmer, A. Sarcevic, V. Fomari, "Panic attacks during discontinuation [withdrawal] of mirtazepine [Remeron]," *Canadian Journal of Psychiatry* 2000;45(65):570–1; C. MacCall, J. Callender, "Mirtazepine [Remeron] withdrawal causing hypomania," *British Journal of Psychiatry* 1999;175:390.

43. *PDR*, 2004, pp. 1658–61.

44. Ibid., pp. 1687–92.

45. N. Michael, A. Erfurth, V. Arolt, "A case report of mania related to discontinuation [withdrawal] of buproprion [Wellbutrin/Zyban] therapy for smoking cessation," *Journal of Clinical Psychiatry* 2004;65(2):277.

46. Price et al., "A comparison of the post-marketing safety of four selective serotonin re-uptake inhibitors including the investigation of symptoms occurring on withdrawal."

47. F. Benazzi, "Venlafaxine [Effexor] withdrawal symptoms," *Canadian Journal of Psychiatry* 1996;41(7):487.

48. Haddad, "Antidepressant discontinuation [withdrawal] syndromes"; M. Lejoyeux, J. Ades, I. Mourad, J. Solomon, S. Dilsaver, "Antidepressant withdrawal syndrome: recognition, prevention and management," *CNS Drugs* 1996;(4):278–92.

49. GlaxoSmithKline, Official product information (product insert) in Italy for Seroxat [the Italian name for Paxil], March 2002, English translation.

50. GlaxoSmithKline, Official product information (product insert) in Switzerland for Deroxat [the Swiss name for Paxil], January 9, 1997, English translation.

51. American Psychiatric Association, *Diagnostic and Statistical Manual of Mental Disorders*, 4th Ed. (Washington D.C.: American Psychiatric Association, 1994), p. 327.

52. Haddad, "The SSRI discontinuation [withdrawal] syndrome"; Black et al., "Selective serotonin reuptake inhibitor discontinuation [withdrawal] syndrome: proposed diagnostic criteria"; Schatzberg et al., "Serotonin reuptake inhibitor discontinuation [withdrawal] syndrome: a hypothetical definition."

53. B. Sadock and V. Sadock, *Kaplan and Sadock's Synopsis of Psychiatry*, 9th Ed., (Philadelphia: Lippincott Williams & Wilkins, 2003), p. 568.

54. Reeves and Pinkofsky, "Lhermitte's sign in paroxetine [Paxil] withdrawal"; S.D. Phillips, "A possible paroxetine [Paxil] withdrawal syndrome," *Ameri-*

can Journal of Psychiatry 1995;152(4):645–6; Farah and Lauer, "Possible venlafaxine [Effexor] withdrawal syndrome."

55. G.M. Strickland, D.W. Hough, "Unilateral facial numbness and visual blurring associated with paroxetine [Paxil] discontinuation [withdrawal]," *Journal of Clinical Psychopharmacology* 2000;20(2):271–2; Rosenbaum and Zajecka, "Clinical management of antidepressant discontinuation [withdrawal]."

56. Rosenbaum and Zajecka, "Clinical management of antidepressant discontinuation [withdrawal]."

57. E. Einbinder, "Fluoxetine [Prozac] withdrawal?" *American Journal of Psychiatry* 1995;152(8):1235.

58. Strickland and Hough, "Unilateral facial numbness and visual blurring associated with paroxetine [Paxil] discontinuation [withdrawal]."

59. Reeves and Pinkofsky, "Lhermitte's sign in paroxetine [Paxil] withdrawal."

60. P.M. Haddad, S. Devarajan, S.M. Dursun, "Antidepressant discontinuation [withdrawal] symptoms presenting as 'stroke,' " *Journal of Psychopharmacology* 2001;15(2):139–41.

61. Schatzberg et al., "Serotonin reuptake inhibitor discontinuation [withdrawal] syndrome."

Chapter 4. How Changing the Dose May Make Patients Suicidal

1. American Psychiatric Association, *Diagnostic and Statistical Manual of Mental Disorders,* 4th Ed. (Washington, DC: American Psychiatric Press, 1994), p. 372.

2. *Physician's Desk Reference (PDR),* (Montvale, NJ: Thomson PDR, 2004), pp. 1292–6.

3. J. Glenmullen, *Prozac Backlash: Overcoming the Dangers of Prozac, Zoloft, Paxil, and Other Antidepressants with Safe, Effective Alternatives* (New York: Simon & Schuster, 2000).

4. http://www.fda.gov/cder/drug/antidepressants/AntidepressantsPHA.htm.

5. C.T. Gualtieri, "Paradoxical effects of fluoxetine [Prozac]," *Journal of Clinical Psychopharmacology* 1991;11:393–4; M.H. Teicher, C.A. Glod, J.O. Cole, "Antidepressant drugs and the emergence of suicidal tendencies," *Drug Safety* 1993;8:186–212.

6. Most of the case reports and research to date on antidepressant-induced suicidality have focused on SSRIs.

7. N. Angier, "Eli Lilly facing million-dollar suits on its antidepressant drug Prozac," *The New York Times,* August 16, 1990, p. B13; A.D. Marcus and W. Lambert, "Eli Lilly to pay costs of doctors sued after they prescribe Prozac," *Wall Street Journal,* June 6, 1991, p. B1; A.D. Marcus, "Prozac firm fights drug's use as defense," *Wall Street Journal,* April 9, 1991, p. B8; M. Mitka, "Drug maker to defend physicians sued over Prozac," *American*

Medical News, June 24, 1991, p. 14; P. Masand, S. Gupta, M. Dewan, "Suicidal ideation related to fluoxetine [Prozac] treatment," *New England Journal of Medicine* 1991;324:420; M.H. Teicher, C. Glod, and J.O. Cole, "Emergence of intense suicidal preoccupation during fluoxetine [Prozac] treatment," *American Journal of Psychiatry* 1990;147:207–10.

8. Masand, Gupta, and Dewan, "Suicidal ideation related to fluoxetine [Prozac] treatment"; Teicher et al., "Emergence of intense suicidal preoccupation during fluoxetine [Prozac] treatment"; K. Dasgupta, "Additional cases of suicidal ideation associated with fluoxetine [Prozac]," *American Journal of Psychiatry* 1990;147:1570; L.A. Papp and J.M. Gorman, "Suicidal preoccupation during fluoxetine [Prozac] treatment," *American Journal of Psychiatry* 1990;147: 1380; J.J. Mann and S. Kapur, "The emergence of suicidal ideation and behavior during antidepressant pharmacotherapy," *Archives of General Psychiatry* 1991;48:1027–33; H. Koizumi, "Fluoxetine [Prozac] and suicidal ideation," *Journal of the American Academy of Child and Adolescent Psychiatry* 1991;30:695; R.A. King, M.A. Riddle, P.B. Chappell, M.T. Hardin, G.M. Anderson, P. Lombroso, L. Scahill, "Emergence of self-destructive phenomena in children and adolescents during fluoxetine [Prozac] treatment," *Journal of the American Academy of Child and Adolescent Psychiatry* 1991;30:179–86; W. Creaney, I. Murray, D. Healy, "Antidepressant [Prozac and Luvox]-induced suicidal ideation," *Human Psychopharmacology* 1991;6:329–32; M.J. Dewan and P. Masand, "Prozac and suicide," *Journal of Family Practice* 1991;33:312; Editorial, "5-HT Blockers [SSRIs] and all that," *Lancet* August 11, 1990, p. 345; A.J. Rothschild and C.A. Locke, "Re-exposure to fluoxetine [Prozac] after serious suicide attempts by three patients: the role of akathisia," *Journal of Clinical Psychiatry* 1991;52:491–3; W.C. Wirshing, T. Van Putten, J. Rosenberg, S. Marder, D. Ames, and T. Hicks-Gray, "Fluoxetine [Prozac], akathisia and suicidality: is there a causal connection?" *Archives of General Psychiatry* 1992;49:580–1; M.S. Hamilton and L.A. Opler; "Akathisia, suicidality, and fluoxetine [Prozac]," *Journal of Clinical Psychiatry* 1992;53:401–6.

9. Internal Eli Lilly memo, "FDA meeting to discuss fluoxetine [Prozac] rechallenge protocol, May 13, 1991," written by James G. Kotsansos on May 15, 1991. Plaintiff's exhibit number 125 in *Susan Forsyth et al. v. Eli Lilly et al.* Case No. 95-00185 ACK, United States District Court for the District of Hawaii.

10. Internal Eli Lilly document. Memo from M.W. Talbott, Director Medical Regulatory Affairs, Eli Lilly and Company to the Food and Drug Administration, Center for Drug Evaluation and Research, Division of Neuropharmacological Drug Products, March 29, 1991. The memo details the study protocol and includes the more sensitive rating scales for assessing suicidality.

11. http://www.fda.gov/cder/drug/antidepressants/AntidepressantsPHA.htm; http://medicines.mhra.gove.uk/ourwork/monitorsafequalmed/safetymessages/ssrioverview_101203.htm; GlaxoSmithKline, "Dear Doctor" Letter,

June 10, 2003, sent to doctors in the United Kingdom; Wyeth, "Dear Health Care Professional" Letter, August 22, 2003; P. Breggin, "Suicidality, violence and mania caused by selective serotonin reuptake inhibitors (SSRIs): a review and analysis," *International Journal of Risk and Safety in Medicine* 2003/ 2004;16:31–49; Declaration of David Healy, M.D., in *Susan Forsyth et al., v. Eli Lilly et al.,* Case No. 95-00185 ACK, United States District Court for the District of Hawaii, pp. 15–6; Teicher, Glod, and Cole, "Antidepressant drugs and the emergence of suicidal tendencies."

12. G.R. Jaimeson and J.H. Wall, "Some psychiatric aspects of suicide," *Psychiatric Quarterly* 1933;7:211–29.

13. M. Y. Agargun, H. Kara, M. Solmaz, "Sleep disturbances and suicidal behavior in patients with major depression," *Journal of Clinical Psychiatry* 1997;58(6):249–51.

14. J. Fawcett, W.A. Scheftner, L. Fogg et al., "Time-related predictors of suicide in major affective disorder," *American Journal of Psychiatry* 1990;147: 1189–94.

15. J. Fawcett, "The detection and consequences of anxiety in clinical depression," *Journal of Clinical Psychiatry* 1997;58(suppl 8):35–40; Fawcett, Scheftner, Fogg et al., "Time-related predictors of suicide in major affective disorder."

16. American Psychiatric Association, *Diagnostic and Statistical Manual of Mental Disorders, 4th Ed.,* pp. 394–5.

17. J. Johnson, M.M. Weissman, G.L. Klerman, "Panic disorder, comorbidity, and suicide attempts," *Archives of General Psychiatry* 1990;47:805–8; M.M. Weissman, G.L. Klerman, J.S. Markowitz, R. Ouellette, "Suicidal ideation and suicide attempts in panic disorder and attacks," *New England Journal of Medicine* 1989;321:1209–14.

18. *PDR,* 2004, pp. 2690–96.

19. T. Van Putten, L.R. Mutalipassi, M.D. Malkin, "Phenothiazine-induced decompensation," *Archives of General Psychiatry* 1974;30:102–5; T. Van Putten, "The many faces of akathisia," *Comprehensive Psychiatry* 1975;16:43–7; T. Van Putten, S.R. Marder, "Behavioral toxicity of antipsychotic drugs," *Journal of Clinical Psychiatry* 1987;48(suppl 9):13–19; T. Van Putten, "Why do schizophrenic patients refuse to take their drugs?" *Archives of General Psychiatry* 1974;31:67–72. Akathisia's association with suicide and violence is well-known from an earlier class of drugs called antipsychotics.

20. J.F. Lipinski, Jr., G. Mallya, P. Zimmerman, and H.G. Pope, "Fluoxetine [Prozac]–induced akathisia: clinical and theoretical implications," *Journal of Clinical Psychiatry* 1989;50:339–42; R.J. Leo, "Movement disorders associated with the serotonin selective reuptake inhibitors," *Journal of Clinical Psychiatry* 1996;57:449–54; Hamilton and Opler, "Akathisia, suicidality, and fluoxetine [Prozac]"; Wirshing et al.,"Fluoxetine [Prozac], akathisia, and suicidality: is there a causal connection?"; Glenmullen, *Prozac Backlash,* pp. 135–86.

21. *PDR,* 2004, pp. 1292–6, 1302–6, 1583–94, 1840–6, 2690–6; *PDR,* 2000,

pp. 3070–3. Note that Pfizer lists "hyperkinesia" as a side effect of Zoloft. Hyperkinesia is another name for akathisia. Pfizer also lists "extrapyramidal symptoms," the family of side effects that includes akathisia.

22. American Psychiatric Association, *Diagnostic and Statistical Manual of Mental Disorders,* 4th Ed., 1994, p. 745.

23. A.F. Schatzberg and C.B. Nemeroff, *Textbook of Psychopharmacology,* 2nd Ed. (Washington, DC: American Psychiatric Press, 1998), p. 939.

24. Van Putten, "The many faces of akathisia"; Van Putten and Marder, "Behavioral toxicity of antipsychotic drugs," Van Putten, "Why do schizophrenic patients refuse to take their drugs?"; Van Putten, Mutalipassi, Malkin, "Phenothiazine-induced decompensation."

25. Van Putten, "The many faces of akathisia."

26. L.B. Kalinowsky, "Appraisal of the 'tranquilizers' [later called "major tranquilizers" or antipsychotics] and their influence on other somatic treatments in psychiatry," *American Journal of Psychiatry* 1958;115:294–300.

27. Hamilton and Opler; "Akathisia, suicidality, and fluoxetine [Prozac]."

28. Glenmullen, *Prozac Backlash,* pp. 135–86.

29. R.M. Lane, "SSRI-Induced extrapyramidal side-effects and akathisia: implications for treatment," *Journal of Psychopharmacology* 1998;12:192–214.

30. W.A. Keckich, "Neuroleptics: Violence as a manifestation of akathisia," *JAMA* 1978;240:2185; E.D. Shaw, J.J. Mann, P.J. Weiden, L.M. Sinsheimer, R.D. Brunn, "A case of suicidal and homicidal ideation and akathisia in a double-blind neuroleptic [major tranquilizer or antipsychotic] crossover study," *Journal of Clinical Psychopharmacology* 1986;6:196–7; J.L. Schulte, "Homicide and suicide associated with akathisia and haloperidol [Haldol]," *American Journal of Forensic Psychiatry,* 1985;6:3–7.

31. Declaration of Jonathan Cole, M.D., in *Miller vs. Pfizer, Inc.,* United States District Court, District of Kansas, April 28, 2000, Case No. 99-2326 KHV.

32. Rothschild and Locke, "Re-exposure to fluoxetine [Prozac] after serious suicide attempts by three patients: the role of akathisia"; Wirshing et al., "Fluoxetine [Prozac], akathisia and suicidality: is there a causal connection?"

33. American Psychiatric Association, *Diagnostic and Statistical Manual of Mental Disorders, 4th Ed.,* pp. 328–38.

34. Ibid., p. 330.

35. *PDR,* 2004, pp. 1292–6, 1302–6, 1583–94, 1658–65, 1687–92, 1840–6, 2389–92, 2690–6, 3413–24; *PDR,* 2000, pp. 849–53, 3070–3. Note that the official information on Wellbutrin uses slightly different phraseology: "activation of psychosis and/or mania."

36. *PDR,* 2004, p. 1659.

37. R.C. Morais, "Prozac nation: is the party over?" *Forbes,* September 6, 2004, pp. 119–24.

38. L. Kowalczyk, "Pfizer unit agrees to $430 million in fines," *Boston Globe,* May 14, 2004.

39. Ibid.
40. Ibid.
41. Ibid.
42. Ibid.
43. D. Healy, *Antidepressant Era* (Cambridge: Harvard University Press, 1991).
44. *PDR,* 2004, pp. 1292–6, 1302–6, 1583–94, 1687–92, 1840–6, 2389–92, 2690–6, 3413–24.
45. P. Breggin, *Talking Back to Prozac* (New York: St. Martin's Press, 1994); P. Breggin, "Suicidality, violence and mania caused by selective serotonin reuptake inhibitors (SSRIs): a review and analysis," *International Journal of Risk and Safety in Medicine* 2003/2004;16:31–49; P. Breggin and D. Cohen, *Your Drug May Be Your Problem* (Cambridge: Perseus Publishing, 1999), p. 126.
46. *PDR,* 2004, pp. 1292–6, 1583–94, 1840–6, 2690–6, 3413–24; *PDR,* 2000, pp. 849–53.
47. T.J. Feurstein and R. Jacksich, "Why do some antidepressants promote suicide?" *Psychopharmacology* 1980;90:422.
48. http://www.fda.gov/cdcr/drug/antidepressants/SSRIlabelChange.htm.
49. Ibid.
50. Ibid.
51. Ibid.

Chapter 5. Worst Offenders

1. J. Glenmullen, *Prozac Backlash: Overcoming the Dangers of Prozac, Zoloft, Paxil, and Other Antidepressants with Safe, Effective Alternatives* (New York: Simon & Schuster, 2000).
2. *Physician's Desk Reference (PDR),* (Montvale, NJ: Thomson PDR, 2004), p. 3417.
3. W.J. Giakas, J.M. Davis, "Intractable withdrawal from venlafaxine [Effexor] treated with fluoxetine [Prozac]," *Psychiatric Annals* 1997;27:85–92; P.M. Haddad, "Antidepressant discontinuation [withdrawal] syndromes," *Drug Safety* 2001;24(3):183–97; G. Parker and J. Blennerhassett, "Withdrawal reactions associated with venlafaxine [Effexor]," *Australia and New Zealand Journal of Psychiatry* 1998;32(2):291–4; A.F. Schatzberg, P. Haddad, E.M. Kaplan, M. Lejoyeux, J.F. Rosenbaum, A.H. Young, J. Zajecka, "Serotonin reuptake inhibitor discontinuation [withdrawal] syndrome: a hypothetical definition. Discontinuation Consensus Panel," *Journal of Clinical Psychiatry* 1997;58(suppl 7):5–10; T. Trenque, D. Piednoir, C. Frances, H. Millart, M.L. Germain, "Reports of withdrawal syndrome with the use of SSRIs: a case/non-case study in the French Pharmacovigilance database," *Pharmacoepidemiology and Drug Safety* 2002 Jun;11(4):281–3.
4. *PDR,* 2004, p. 3424.
5. N.J. Coupland, C.J. Bell, J.P. Potokar, "Serotonin reuptake inhibitor with-

2

drawal," *Journal of Psychopharmacology* 1996;16(5):356–62; R.M. Lane, "Withdrawal symptoms after discontinuation of selective serotonin reuptake inhibitors (SSRIs)," *Journal of Serotonin Research*, 1996;3:75–83; P. Haddad, "The SSRI discontinuation [withdrawal] syndrome," *Journal of Psychopharmacology* 1998;12(3):305–13; C. Thompson, "Discontinuation [Withdrawal] of antidepressant therapy; emerging complications and their relevance," *Journal of Clinical Psychiatry* 1998;59(10):541–8.

6. E. Richelson, "Pharmacology of antidepressants," *Mayo Clinic Proceedings* 2001;76:511–27; Lane, "Withdrawal symptoms after discontinuation of selective serotonin reuptake inhibitors (SSRIs)"; A.F. Schatzberg, P. Haddad, E.M. Kaplan, M. Lejoyeux, J.F. Rosenbaum, A.H. Young, J. Zajecka, "Possible biological mechanisms of the serotonin reuptake inhibitor discontinuation [withdrawal] syndrome. Discontinuation Consensus Panel," *Journal of Clinical Psychiatry* 1997;58(suppl 7):23–7.

7. K.P. Lesch, C.S. Aulakh, B.L. Wolozin, T.J. Tolliver, J.L. Hill, D.L. Murphy, "Regional brain expression of serotonin transporter mRNA and its regulation by reuptake inhibiting antidepressants," *Molecular Brain Research* 1993;73: 31–5; Glenmullen, *Prozac Backlash*, p. 94.

8. N.J. Keuthen, P. Cyr, J.A. Ricciardi, W.E. Minichiello, M.L. Buttolph, M.A. Jenike, "Medication withdrawal symptoms in obsessive-compulsive disorder patients treated with paroxetine [Paxil]," *Journal of Clinical Psychopharmacology* 1994;14(3):206–7; Haddad, "The SSRI discontinuation [withdrawal] syndrome"; Haddad, "Antidepressant discontinuation [withdrawal] syndromes."

9. Lane, "Withdrawal symptoms after discontinuation of selective serotonin reuptake inhibitors (SSRIs)"; Haddad, "Antidepressant discontinuation [withdrawal] syndromes."

10. The half-lives are taken from the pharmaceutical companies' official information on the drugs in the *PDR*, 2004. The half-lives given in Table 5.1 are the half-lives of the drugs and do not include the half-lives of any active metabolites. Metabolites are intermediary molecules in the series of steps, or transformations, by which the liver inactivates a drug. Some metabolites are "active," meaning they have some of the same effect as the original drug. Metabolites vary in how active they are, a subject that becomes too technical for the discussion here. Factoring in the half-lives of active metabolites would not significantly alter the conclusions reached in the discussion of Table 5.1. For example, Effexor has an active metabolite, but its half-life is only 11 hours, still shorter than the other antidepressants. Zoloft has an active metabolite, but according to Pfizer it is substantially less active than Zoloft itself. Prozac has an active metabolite with an even longer half-life (9.3 days) than Prozac itself. But Prozac is already the longest-acting antidepressant in Table 5.1. Ninety percent of an antidepressant is eliminated after five half-lives have elapsed. See: Richelson, "Pharmacology of antidepressants." Autoinhibition of metabo-

lism and nonlinear elimination kinetics are two additional pharmacokinetic properties that affect a drug's likelihood of causing withdrawal reactions. But, these factors are too technical for the discussion here and would not significantly alter the conclusions reached in the discussion of Table 5.1.

11. M. Fava, R. Mulroy, J. Alpert, A.A. Nierenberg, J.F. Rosenbaum, "Emergence of adverse events following discontinuation [withdrawal] of treatment with extended-release venlafaxine [Effexor]," *American Journal of Psychiatry* 1997; 154(12):1760–2.

12. J.F. Rosenbaum, M. Fava, S.L. Hoog, R.C. Ascroft, W.B. Krebs, "Selective serotonin reuptake inhibitor discontinuation [withdrawal] syndrome: a randomized clinical trial," *Biological Psychiatry* 1998;44(2):77–87; Fava et al., "Emergence of adverse events following discontinuation [withdrawal] of treatment with extended-release venlafaxine [Effexor]."

13. Haddad, "Antidepressant discontinuation [withdrawal] syndromes."

14. Parker and Blennerhassett, "Withdrawal reactions associated with venlafaxine [Effexor]."

15. *PDR*, 2004, p. 1588.

16. B. Pollock, "Discontinuation [Withdrawal] symptoms and SSRIs," *Journal of Clinical Psychiatry* 1998;59(10):535–6; Haddad, "Antidepressant discontinuation [withdrawal] syndromes"; M.M. Stahl, M. Lindquist, M. Pettersson, I.R. Edwards, J.H. Sanderson, N.F. Taylor, A.P. Fletcher, J.S. Schou, "Withdrawal reactions with selective serotonin re-uptake inhibitors as reported to the WHO system," *European Journal of Clinical Pharmacology* 1997;53(3–4):163–9.

17. Ibid.

18. Rosenbaum et al., "Selective serotonin reuptake inhibitor discontinuation [withdrawal] syndrome."

19. A separate study of Prozac withdrawal reactions is sometimes cited as addressing this problem. (See: J. Zajecka, J. Fawcett, J. Amsterdam, F. Quitkin, F. Reimherr, J. Rosenbaum, D. Michelson, C. Beasley, "Safety of abrupt discontinuation [withdrawal] of fluoxetine [Prozac]: a randomized, placebo-controlled study," *Journal of Clinical Psychopharmacology* 1998;18(3):193–7.) In the study, patients who had stopped 20 milligrams a day of Prozac were monitored for eight days. However, the patients were not systematically asked about withdrawal symptoms, as they were in the study comparing Prozac, Zoloft, and Paxil, where a checklist of withdrawal symptoms was used. Instead, patients were evaluated with "open-ended questioning about general well-being and problems with medication." Such open-ended questions are well known to be much less sensitive in picking up withdrawal reactions than is systematically inquiring about specific withdrawal symptoms, and well known to detect much lower rates of withdrawal reactions. Because of this and other methodological problems, the study did not adequately resolve the issue regarding Prozac withdrawal reactions.

20. Pollock, "Discontinuation [Withdrawal] symptoms and SSRIs."

21. S.M. Stahl, "Not so selective serotonin reuptake inhibitors," *Journal of Clini-*

cal Psychiatry 1998;59:343–44; E. Richelson, "Pharmacology of antidepressants."

22. Glenmullen, *Prozac Backlash,* pp. 195–203.
23. C. O'Brien, "Drug firm to drop non-addiction claim," *Irish Times,* May 10, 2003, p. 4.
24. Glenmullen, *Prozac Backlash,* pp. 48–51.
25. Richelson, "Pharmacology of antidepressants."
26. Schatzberg et al., "Possible biological mechanisms of the serotonin reuptake inhibitor discontinuation [withdrawal] syndrome."
27. IMS HEALTH, "IMS HEALTH reports 10 percent growth in 2000 audited global total pharmaceutical sales to $317.2 billion," March 6, 2001; IMS HEALTH, "IMS HEALTH reports 8 percent constant dollar growth in 2002 audited global pharmaceutical sales to 400.6 billion," February 25, 2003.
28. D. Kirkpatrick, "Inside the happiness business," *New York Magazine,* May 15, 2000, pp. 37–43.
29. SmithKlineBeecham [now GlaxoSmithKline], "Paxil (paroxetine): Patient Question & Answer Guide," July 1997; GlaxoSmithKline, "Generalized Anxiety Disorder," April 2001. The phrase "non-habit forming" was used in television advertisements.

Chapter 6. The 5-Step Antidepressant Tapering Program

1. L.F. Koopowitz and M. Berk, "Paroxetine [Paxil]-induced withdrawal effects," *Human Psychopharmacology* 1995;10:147–8.
2. W.J. Giakas and J.M. Davis, "Intractable withdrawal from venlafaxine [Effexor] treated with fluoxetine [Prozac]," *Psychiatric Annals* 1997;27:85–92; S.L. Rauch, R.L. O'Sullivan, M.A. Jenike, "Open treatment of obsessive-compulsive disorder with venlafaxine [Effexor]: a series of ten cases," *Journal of Clinical Psychopharmacology* 1996;16(1):81–4; S.D. Phillips, "A possible paroxetine [Paxil] withdrawal syndrome," *American Journal of Psychiatry* 1995;152(4):645–6; S. Nuss, C.R. Kincaid, "Serotonin discontinuation [withdrawal] syndrome: does it really exist?" *West Virginia Medical Journal* 2000;96(2):405–7; N.J. Keuthen, P. Cyr, J.A. Ricciardi, W.E. Minichiello, M.L. Buttolph, M.A. Jenike, "Medication withdrawal symptoms in obsessive-compulsive disorder patients treated with paroxetine [Paxil]," *Journal of Clinical Psychopharmacology* 1994;14(3):206–7.
3. J.S. Price, P.C. Waller, S.M. Wood, A.V. MacKay, "A comparison of the postmarketing safety of four selective serotonin re-uptake inhibitors including the investigation of symptoms occurring on withdrawal," *British Journal of Clinical Pharmacology* 1996;42(6):757–63.
4. J.O. Schechter, "Treatment of disequilibrium and nausea in the SRI discontinuation [withdrawal] syndrome," *Journal of Clinical Psychiatry* 1998;59(8): 431–2.

Chapter 7. Step 1: Evaluating Whether You Are Ready

1. P. Kramer, *Listening to Prozac* (New York: Viking, 1993) pp. xvi–xix.
2. M. Babyak, J. Blumenthal, S. Herman, P. Khatri, M. Doraiswamy, K. Moore, E. Craighead, T. Baldewicz, R. Krishnan, "Exercise treatment for major depression: maintenance of therapeutic benefit at 10 months," *Psychosomatic Medicine* 2000;62:633–8; J. Blumenthal, M. Babyak, K. Moore, E. Craighead, S. Herman, P. Khatri, R. Waugh, M. Napolitano, M. Doraiswamy, R. Krishnan, "Effects of exercise training on older patients with major depression," *Archives of Internal Medicine* 1999;159:2349–56.
3. C. O'Brien, "Drug firm to drop non-addiction claim," *Irish Times,* May 10, 2003, p. 4.
4. J. Glenmullen, *Prozac Backlash: Overcoming the Dangers of Prozac, Zoloft, Paxil, and Other Antidepressants with Safe, Effective Alternatives* (New York: Simon & Schuster, 2000), pp. 198–201.
5. J.A. Egeland, D.S. Gerhard, D.L. Pauls, J.N. Sussex, K.K. Kidd, C.R. Allen, A.M. Hostetter, D.E. Housman, "Bipolar affective disorders linked to DNA markers on chromosome 11," *Nature* 1987;325:783–7. The retraction in *Nature* appeared almost two years after publication of the original study: J.R. Kelsoe, E.I. Ginns, J.A. Egeland, D.S. Gerhard, A.M. Goldstein, S.J. Bale, D.L. Pauls, R.T. Long, K.K. Kidd, G. Conte, D.E. Housman, S.M. Paul, "Reevaluation of the linkage relationship between chromosome 11p loci and the gene for bipolar affective disorder in the Old Order Amish," *Nature* 1989;342:238–43. See also: R. Lewontin, "The dream of the human genome," *New York Review of Books,* May 28, 1992.
6. Glenmullen, *Prozac Backlash,* pp. 192–3.
7. American Psychiatric Association, *Diagnostic and Statistical Manual of Mental Disorders,* 4th Ed. (Washington D.C.: American Psychiatric Association, 1994), pp. 339–45.
8. D. Healy, *Let Them Eat Prozac* (Toronto: James Lorimer, 2003), p. 401.

Chapter 8. Step 2: Making the Initial Dosage Reductions

1. R.S. Diler, L. Tamam, A. Avci, "Withdrawal symptoms associated with paroxetine [Paxil] discontinuation in a nine-year-old boy," *Journal of Clinical Psychopharmacology* 2000;20(5):586–7.
2. *Physician's Desk Reference (PDR),* (Montvale, NJ: Thomson PDR, 2004), pp. 1658–65.
3. Ibid., pp. 1840–6.
4. Eli Lilly and Company, "Sarafem: fluoxetine [Prozac] hydrochloride," Patient information summary, January 2004.
5. *PDR,* 2004, pp. 2389–92.

Chapter 9. Step 3: Monitoring Withdrawal Symptoms

1. D. Michelson, M. Fava, J. Amsterdam, J. Apter, P. Londborg, R. Tamura, R.G. Tepner, "Interruption of selective serotonin reuptake inhibitor treatment. Double-blind, placebo-controlled trial," *British Journal of Psychiatry* 2000;176:363–8; N.J. Coupland, C.J. Bell, J.P. Potokar, "Serotonin reuptake inhibitor withdrawal," *Journal of Clinical Psychopharmacology* 1996;16(5):356–62; S. Nuss, C.R. Kincaid, "Serotonin discontinuation [withdrawal] syndrome: does it really exist?" *West Virginia Medical Journal* 2000;96(2):405–7; M. Lejoyeux, J. Ades, I. Mourad, J. Solomon, S. Dilsaver, "Antidepressant withdrawal syndrome: recognition, prevention and management," *CNS Drugs* 1996;4:278–92; M. Lejoyeux, J. Ades, "Antidepressant discontinuation [withdrawal]: a review of the literature," *Journal of Clinical Psychiatry* 1997;58(suppl 7):11–16; J.F. Rosenbaum, M. Fava, S.L. Hoog, R.C. Ascroft, W.B. Krebs, "Selective serotonin reuptake inhibitor discontinuation [withdrawal] syndrome: a randomized clinical trial," *Biological Psychiatry* 1998;44(2):77–87.

2. R. Judge, M.G. Parry, D. Quail, J.G. Jacobson, "Discontinuation [Withdrawal] symptoms: comparison of brief interruption in fluoxetine [Prozac] and paroxetine [Paxil] treatment," *International Clinical Psychopharmacology* 2002;17(5):217–25; Rosenbaum et al., "Selective serotonin reuptake inhibitor discontinuation [withdrawal] syndrome."

3. Coupland et al., "Serotonin reuptake inhibitor withdrawal"; S. Oehrberg, P.E. Christiansen, K. Behnke, A.L. Borup, B. Severin, J. Soegaard, H. Calberg, R. Judge, J.K. Ohrstrom, P.M. Manniche, "Paroxetine [Paxil] in the treatment of panic disorder. A randomised, double-blind, placebo-controlled study," *British Journal of Psychiatry* 1995;167(3):374–9.

4. K. Black, C. Shea, S. Dursun, S. Kutcher, "Selective serotonin reuptake inhibitor discontinuation [withdrawal] syndrome: proposed diagnostic criteria," *Journal of Psychiatry and Neuroscience* 2000;25(3):255–61; Rosenbaum et al., "Selective serotonin reuptake inhibitor discontinuation [withdrawal] syndrome"; F. Bogetto, S. Bellino, R.B. Revello, L. Patria, "Discontinuation [Withdrawal] syndrome in dysthymic patients treated with selective serotonin reuptake inhibitors: a clinical investigation," *CNS Drugs* 2002;16(4):273–83.

5. L. Frost, S. Lal, "Shock-like sensations after discontinuation [withdrawal] of selective serotonin reuptake inhibitors," *American Journal of Psychiatry* 1995;152(5):810; J.S. Price, P.C. Waller, S.M. Wood, A.V. MacKay, "A comparison of the post-marketing safety of four selective serotonin re-uptake inhibitors including the investigation of symptoms occurring on withdrawal," *British Journal of Psychiatry* 1996;42(6):757–63; Black et al., "Selective serotonin reuptake inhibitor discontinuation [withdrawal] syndrome"; C.S. Berlin, "Fluoxetine [Prozac] withdrawal symptoms," *Journal of Clinical Psychiatry* 1996;57(2):93–4.

6. Rosenbaum et al., "Selective serotonin reuptake inhibitor discontinuation [withdrawal] syndrome"; M. Fava, R. Mulroy, J. Alpert, A.A. Nierenberg, J.F. Rosenbaum, "Emergence of adverse events following discontinuation [withdrawal] of treatment with extended-release venlafaxine [Effexor]," *American Journal of Psychiatry* 1997;154(12):1760–2.

7. J. Winkelman, C. Dorsey, S. Cunningham et al., "Fluoxetine [Prozac] produces persistent rapid eye movements in non-REM sleep," *Sleep Research* 1992;21:78; R. Armitage, M. Trivedi, A.J. Rush, "Fluoxetine [Prozac] and oculomotor activity during sleep in depressed patients," *Neuropsychopharmacology* 1995;12(2):159–65; C.H. Schneck, M.W. Mahowald, S.W. Kim et al. "Prominent eye movements during NREM sleep and REM sleep behavior disorder associated with fluoxetine [Prozac] treatment of depression and obsessive-compulsive disorder," *Sleep* 1992;15(3)226–35.

Chapter 12. Tapering Children Off Antidepressants

1. *Physician's Desk Reference (PDR)*, (Montvale, NJ: Thomson PDR, 2004), pp. 3413–24.

2. R.S. Diler, L. Tamam, A. Avci, "Withdrawal symptoms associated with paroxetine [Paxil] discontinuation [withdrawal] in a nine-year-old boy," *Journal of Clinical Psychopharmacology* 2000;20(5):586–7.

3. J. Glenmullen, *Prozac Backlash: Overcoming the Dangers of Prozac, Zoloft, Paxil, and Other Antidepressants with Safe, Effective Alternatives* (New York: Simon & Schuster, 2000).

4. http://medicines.mhra.gove.uk/ourwork/monitorsafequalmed/safetymessages/ssrioverview_101203.htm; http://www.fda.gov/cder/drug/antidepressants/Antidepressants PHA.htm.

5. S. Boseley, "Drugs for depressed children banned," *The Guardian*, December 10, 2003.

6. *Panorama*, "The Secrets of Seroxat [Paxil]," The British Broadcasting Company (BBC), October 13, 2002; *Panorama*, "Seroxat [Paxil]: Emails from the Edge," The British Broadcasting Company (BBC), May 11, 2003.

7. http://medicines.mhra.gove.uk/ourwork/monitorsafequalmed/safetymessages/ssrioverview_101203.htm.

8. C. Whittington, T. Kendall, P. Fonagy, D. Cottrell, A. Cotgrove, E. Boddington, "Selective serotonin reuptake inhibitors in childhood depression: systematic review of published versus unpublished data," *Lancet* 2004;363:1335; Editorial, "Depressing research," *Lancet* 2004;363:1335.

9. J.N. Jureidini, C.J. Doeke, P.R. Mansfield, M.M. Haby, D.B. Menkes, and A.L. Tonkin, "Efficacy and safety of antidepressants for children and adolescents," *British Medical Journal* 2004;328:879–83.

10. C. Johnson, "Suicide warning ordered on drugs: antidepressant risk seen in youth," *Boston Globe*, October 16, 2004, p. A1; E. Shogren, "FDA orders

depression drug warning; antidepressant labels will have to carry a prominent
alert about the risk of suicidal thought and behavior in children and teens,"
Los Angeles Times, October 16, 2004, p. A8; G. Harris, "FDA toughens warning on antidepressant drugs," *New York Times,* October 16, 2004, p. A9.

11. T.J. Moore, "Medical use of antidepressant drugs in children and adults:
1998–2001," January 26, 2004.

12. National Center for Health Statistics, 2001 NAMCS Micro-Data File Documentation, *National Center for Health Statistics* 2003 December; National
Center for Health Statistics, 2001 NHAMCS Micro-Data File Documentation, *National Center for Health Statistics* 2003 December.

13. *PDR,* 2004, pp. 1840–6.

14. Ibid., pp. 1840–6, 2690–6; *Physician's Desk Reference (PDR)* (Montvale, NJ:
Thomson PDR, 2000), pp. 3070–3.

15. S. Vedantam, "Child antidepressant warning is urged: panel's recommendation to FDA comes as use of medicine has soared," *The Washington Post,* September 15, 2004, p. A02.

16. Ibid.

17. Andrew D. Mosholder, "Suicidality in pediatric clinical trials with Paxil and
other antidepressant drugs: Follow up to 9-2-03 consult," FDA memo, February 18, 2004, p. 21.

18. Andrew D. Mosholder, "Suicidality in pediatric clinical trials of antidepressant drugs: Comparison between previous analyses and Columbia University
classification," FDA memo, August 16, 2004, p. 6.

Afterword

1. *Physician's Desk Reference (PDR),* (Montvale, NJ: Thomson PDR, 1997), pp.
2681–6. Paxil "withdrawal syndrome" is listed under nervous system side effects on p. 2686. In 2001, GlaxoSmithKline added sections on frequent Paxil
"discontinuation" symptoms (see: *PDR,* 2004, pp. 1585 and 1589) but left the
statement that Paxil rarely causes a "withdrawal syndrome." See Chapter 2 for
a discussion of the euphemism "antidepressant discontinuation syndrome"
for antidepressant withdrawal reactions.

2. *PDR,* 1997, pp. 2051–3. Zoloft "withdrawal syndrome" is listed under psychiatric side effects on page 2053.

3. *PDR,* 2004, p. 1588.

4. J.F. Rosenbaum, M. Fava, S.L. Hoog, R.C. Ascroft, W.B. Krebs, "Selective
serotonin reuptake inhibitor discontinuation [withdrawal] syndrome: a randomized clinical trial," *Biological Psychiatry* 1998;44(2):77–87.

5. J. Glenmullen, *Prozac Backlash: Overcoming the Dangers of Prozac, Zoloft,
Paxil, and Other Antidepressants with Safe, Effective Alternatives* (New York:
Simon & Schuster, 2000), pp. 20–24.

6. *PDR,* 1997, pp. 2681–6 and 2051–3.

7. A. Weil, "The new politics of coca," *The New Yorker*, May 15, 1995, pp. 70–80.

8. Ibid.

9. T.J. Moore, *Prescription for Disaster* (New York: Simon & Schuster, 1998), p. 88.

10. J.G. Hardman and L.E. Limbird, Eds., *Goodman & Gilman's The Pharmacological Basis of Therapeutics*, 10th Edition (New York: McGraw-Hill, 2001), pp. 634–6.

11. *PDR*, 2004, pp. 1840–6.

12. E. Richelson, "Pharmacology of antidepressants," *Mayo Clinic Proceedings* 2001;76:511–27.

13. *PDR*, 2004, pp. 3413–24.

14. Richelson, "Pharmacology of antidepressants."

15. Hardman and Limbird, Eds., *Goodman & Gilman's The Pharmacological Basis of Therapeutics*, pp. 634–6.

16. Richelson, "Pharmacology of antidepressants."

17. Ibid. Richelson coins the acronym "SNUB" for these "super neurotransmitter uptake [i.e., reuptake] blockers [i.e., inhibitors]."

18. Glenmullen, *Prozac Backlash*, p. 20.

19. Moore, *Prescription for Disaster*, p. 17.

20. D.A. Kessler, "Introducing MedWatch," *Journal of the American Medical Association* 1993;269:2765–68.

21. P.J. Walker, J.O. Cole, E.A. Garnder, A.R. Hughs, J.A. Johnston, S.R. Batey, C.G. Lineberry, "Improvement in fluoxetine [Prozac]-associated sexual dysfunction in patients switched to buproprion [Wellbutrin]," *Journal of Clinical Psychiatry* 1993;54:459–65; R.T. Segraves, K.B. Segraves, C.N. Bubna, "Sexual function in patients taking buproprion [Wellbutrin] sustained release," *Journal of Psychiatry* 1995;56:374; A. Feiger, A. Kiev, R.K. Shirvastava, P.G. Wisselink, C.S. Wilcox, "Nefazodone [Serzone] versus sertraline [Zoloft] in outpatients with major depression: focus on efficacy, tolerability, and effects on sexual function and satisfaction," *Journal of Clinical Psychiatry* 1996; 57(suppl 2):53–62; J. Brody, Personal Health column, *The New York Times*, May 15, 1996, p. C8.

22. R. Jacobsen, "Bristol drug seen having fewer sexual side effects," Reuters Financials Service, New York newsdesk, May 8, 1996.

23. J. Brody, "Wonder drugs to brighten moods can dim libido: but there are solutions available to those left sexually bereft," *Star Tribune* (Minneapolis), May 19, 1996, p. E3; Brody, Personal Health column; S.G. Boodman, "Some antidepressants put hex on sex," *Des Moines* Register, July 22, 1996, Today section, p. 3; S.G. Boodman, "Antidepressants can interfere with sex: studies compare problems with patients taking Serzone and Zoloft," *Washington Post*, May 21, 1996; D.M. Rios, "Women urged to talk about antidepressants' effect on sex," *Austin American-Statesman*, November 26, 1997, p. D1; J.

Brody, "Sexual side effects of antidepressants," *International Herald Tribune*, May 16, 1996, Feature section.

24. Rosenbaum et al., "Selective serotonin reuptake inhibitor discontinuation [withdrawal] syndrome: a randomized clinical trial."
25. *Journal of Clinical Psychiatry*, 1997;58(suppl 7). See inside cover for statement of Lilly sponsorship. See additional discussion of the euphemism "antidepressant discontinuation syndrome" in Chapter 2.
26. A.F. Schatzberg, P. Haddad, E.M. Kaplan, M. Lejoyeux, J.F. Rosenbaum, A.H. Young, and J. Zajecka, "Serotonin reuptake inhibitor discontinuation [withdrawal] syndrome: hypothetical definition," *Journal of Clinical Psychiatry*, 1997;58(suppl 7):5–10. See Dr. Jerrold Rosenbaum's comments in the discussion at the end of the paper.
27. B. Pollock, "Discontinuation [Withdrawal] symptoms and SSRIs," *Journal of Clinical Psychiatry* 1998;59(10):535–6; P.M. Haddad, "Antidepressant discontinuation [withdrawal] syndromes," *Drug Safety* 2001;24(3):183–97; M.M. Stahl, M. Lindquist, M. Pettersson, I.R. Edwards, J.H. Sanderson, N.F. Taylor, A.P. Fletcher, J.S. Schou, "Withdrawal reactions with selective serotonin re-uptake inhibitors as reported to the WHO system," *European Journal of Clinical Pharmacology* 1997;53(3–4):163–9.
28. Glenmullen, *Prozac Backlash*, pp. 130–4.
29. Pollock, "Discontinuation [Withdrawal] symptoms and SSRIs."
30. J. Zajecka, J. Fawcett, J. Amsterdam, F. Quitkin, F. Reimherr, J. Rosenbaum, D. Michelson, C. Beasley, "Safety of abrupt discontinuation [withdrawal] of fluoxetine [Prozac]: a randomized, placebo-controlled study," *Journal of Clinical Psychopharmacology* 1998;18(3):193–7.
31. Ibid.
32. Rosenbaum et al., "Selective serotonin reuptake inhibitor discontinuation [withdrawal] syndrome."
33. Zajecka et al., "Safety of abrupt discontinuation [withdrawal] of fluoxetine [Prozac]."
34. Schatzberg et al., "Serotonin reuptake inhibitor [Prozac-type drug] discontinuation [withdrawal] syndrome,"
35. Ibid. See discussion at the end of the paper. This is one of eight papers published by the participants at the Lilly-funded meeting of "experts" to discuss the "antidepressant discontinuation syndrome." In addition to supporting the private meeting at a resort in Phoenix, Arizona, Lilly funded mailing the eight academic papers to doctors across the country. In the discussion following the paper, Rosenbaum announces the Lilly-funded research that was already underway.
36. Associated Press, "Shannon widow sues drug company," *Variety*, January 30, 1991; N. Angier, "Suicidal behavior tied again to drug," *The New York Times*, February 7, 1991, p. B15; A.D. Marcus, "Murder trials introduce Prozac defense," *Wall Street Journal*, February 7, 1991, p. B1; A.D. Marcus and W. Lam-

bert, "Eli Lilly to pay costs of doctors sued after they prescribe Prozac," *Wall Street Journal,* June 6, 1991, p. B5; A.D. Marcus, "Prozac firm fights drug's use as defense," *Wall Street Journal,* April 9, 1991, p. B8; M. Mitka, "Drug maker to defend physicians sued over Prozac," *American Medical News,* June 24, 1991, p. 14.

37. M. Fava and J. Rosenbaum, "Suicidality and fluoxetine [Prozac]: is there a relationship?" *Journal of Clinical Psychiatry* 1991;52:108–11.

38. C.M. Beasley, B.E. Dornseif, J.C. Bosomworth, M.E. Sayler, A.H. Rampey, J.H. Heiligenstein, V.L. Thompson, D.J. Murphy, and D.N. Masica, "Fluoxetine [Prozac] and suicide: a meta-analysis of controlled trials of treatment for depression," *British Medical Journal* 1991;303:685–92.

39. L.R. Garnett, "Prozac Revisited: As drug gets remade, concerns about suicides surface," *Boston Sunday Globe,* May 7, 2000, p. A1.

40. D.J. Graham, Internal FDA memo, September 11, 1990, on the subject of Sponsor's [Eli Lilly's] ADR submission on fluoxetine [Prozac] dated July 17, 1990. Department of Health and Human Services, Public Health Service, Food and Drug Administration, Center for Drug Evaluation and Research, Rockville, Maryland. Obtained through the Freedom of Information Act; M.H. Teicher, C.A. Glod, and J.O. Cole, "Antidepressant drugs and the emergence of suicidal tendencies," *Drug Safety* 1993;8:186–212 (see p. 200); Declaration of David Healy, M.D., in *Susan Forsyth et al. v. Eli Lilly et al.* Case No. 95-00185 ACK, United States District Court for the District of Hawaii (see pp. 20–28).

41. Glenmullen, *Prozac Backlash,* pp. 135–86 and notes 54 and 61 on p. 361.

42. Rosenbaum et al., "Selective serotonin reuptake inhibitor discontinuation [withdrawal] syndrome."

43. J.S. Price, P.C. Waller, S.M. Wood, A.V. MacKay, "A comparison of the post-marketing safety of four selective serotonin re-uptake inhibitors including the investigation of symptoms occurring on withdrawal," *British Journal of Clinical Pharmacology* 1996;42(6):757–63.

44. J.F. Rosenbaum and J. Zajecka, "Clinical management of antidepressant discontinuation [withdrawal]," *Journal of Clinical Psychiatry,* 1997;58(suppl 7):37–40.

45. Schatzberg et al., "Serotonin reuptake inhibitor discontinuation [withdrawal] syndrome." See discussion at the end of the paper.

46. Rosenbaum and Zajecka, "Clinical management of antidepressant discontinuation [withdrawal]."

47. Ibid.

48. S. Fried, "Addicted to anti-depressants? The controversy over a pill millions of us are taking," *Glamour,* April 2003, pp. 178–80, 262.

49. M. Duenwald, "How to stop depression medications: very slowly," *The New York Times,* May 25, 2004, Science section.

50. SmithKlineBeecham (which later merged and became GlaxoSmithKline)

memo to the Paxil Selling Team entitled "Discontinuation Syndrome," May 1, 1997.

51. SmithKlineBeecham (which later merged and became GlaxoSmithKline) "Business Plan Guide: A marketing/sales guide to help you tailor your territory business plan," Cycle 2, 1997: December 1, 1997–May 31, 1998.
52. Ruder Finn memo entitled "Discontinuation," June 5, 1997.
53. Pollock, "Discontinuation [Withdrawal] symptoms and SSRIs."
54. Disclosure statements of Dr. Bruce Pollock in the *Journal of Clinical Psychiatry*'s June 2003 CME Info Pack "Treating Aggressive Behavior in the Elderly" and the article "Risk factors for falls during treatment of late-life depression," *Journal of Clinical Psychiatry* 2002;63:936–41.
55. SmithKlineBeecham (which later merged and became GlaxoSmithKline) report on Paxil "Safety Review of Discontinuation [Withdrawal] Symptoms" by Lisa Howell, Tamara Pedgrift, Julie Nash, Dr. R.W. Morris, and Dr. R. Kumar, March 1997; SmithKlineBeecham (which later merged and became GlaxoSmithKline) "Business Plan Guide."
56. SmithKlineBeecham (which later merged and became GlaxoSmithKline) "Business Plan Guide." The "Business Plan Guide" refers to a prescription-event monitoring study done by the Drug Surveillance Research Unit in the United Kingdom, but does not provide a citation for the study. Prescription-event monitoring refers to spontaneous reports by doctors of side effects of drugs once they are released on the market. Because the reports are not systematic, prescription-event monitoring is not a rigorous way of assessing the relative incidence of drug side effects. Early prescription-event monitoring may not have shown differences in the incidence of withdrawal reactions among SSRIs, but by 1997 (the date of the "Business Plan Guide"), side effect reports in the U.K. were showing a higher incidence for Paxil (see: J.S. Price, P.C. Waller, S.M. Wood, A.V. MacKay, "A comparison of the post-marketing safety of four selective serotonin re-uptake inhibitors including the investigation of symptoms occurring on withdrawal," *British Journal of Clinical Pharmacology* 1996;42(6):757–63). Indeed, by 1997 numerous published reports had established a higher incidence for Paxil and other SSRIs with short half-lives.
57. SmithKlineBeecham (which later merged and became GlaxoSmithKline) company sales training guide.
58. SmithKlineBeecham (which later merged and became GlaxoSmithKline) "Business Plan Guide."
59. GlaxoSmithKline, "ACES: A Continuing Education System. Module III. Paxil."
60. SmithKlineBeecham (which later merged and became GlaxoSmithKline) report on Paxil "Safety Review of Discontinuation [Withdrawal] Symptoms."
61. GlaxoSmithKline guide entitled "Central Strategy," 1997.
62. SmithKlineBeecham (which later merged and became GlaxoSmithKline)

transmittal memo entitled "Paroxetine [Paxil]—discontinuation [withdrawal] symptoms," October 29, 1996.

63. GlaxoSmithKline guide entitled "Central Strategy."

64. SmithKlineBeecham (which later merged and became GlaxoSmithKline) memo to the Paxil Selling Team entitled "Discontinuation [Withdrawal] Syndrome."

65. M. Angell, "Is academic medicine for sale?" Editorial, *New England Journal of Medicine* 2000;342:1516–18.

66. C. Whittington, T. Kendall, P. Fonagy, D. Cottrell, A. Cotgrove, E. Boddington, "Selective serotonin reuptake inhibitors in childhood depression: systematic review of published versus unpublished data, *Lancet* 2004;363:1335; Editorial, "Depressing research," *Lancet* 2004;363:1335; J. Jureidini, C.J. Doecke, P.R. Mansfield, M.M. Haby, D.B. Menkes, A.L. Tonkin, "Efficacy and safety of antidepressants for children and adolescents," *British Medical Journal* 2004;328:879–83; S. Brownlee," Doctors without borders: why you can't trust medical journals anymore," *The Washington Monthly*, April 2004, pp. 38–43; L. Kowalczyk, "Pfizer unit agrees to $430 million in fines," *Boston Globe,* May 14, 2004.

67. G. Harris, "New York State official sues drug maker over test data: Glaxo challenged in the use of Paxil for children," *The New York Times,* June 3, 2004, p. A1; B. Martinez, "Spitzer charges Glaxo concealed Paxil data," *Wall Street Journal,* June 3, 2004, p. B1.

68. Kowalczyk, "Pfizer unit agrees to $430 million in fines."

69. N. Angier, "Eli Lilly facing million-dollar suits on its antidepressant drug Prozac," *The New York Times,* August 16, 1990, p. B13; Reuters, "Warning on suicide in Prozac use is sought," *The New York Times,* May 24, 1991; Public Citizen's petition for revision of fluoxetine [Prozac] labeling, Memorandum from Dr. Sidney Wolfe and Dr. Ida Hellander of the Public Citizen Health Research Group to Dr. David Kessler, Commissioner of the Food and Drug Administration, May 23, 1991.

70. Conflict of Interest Statement for the Psychopharmacologic Drugs Advisory Committee, Department of Health and Human Services, Public Health Service, Food and Drug Administration, Rockville, Maryland, September 20, 1991. Obtained through the Freedom of Information Act.

71. Ibid.

72. Transcript of the Food and Drug Administration, Psychopharmacological Drugs Advisory Committee, Department of Health and Human Services, Public Health Service, Food and Drug Administration, Rockville, Maryland, September 20, 1991, p. 331. Obtained through the Freedom of Information Act.

73. Internal Eli Lilly memo, "FDA meeting to discuss fluoxetine [Prozac] rechallenge protocol, May 13, 1991," written by James G. Kotsansos on May 15, 1991. Plaintiff's exhibit number 125 in *Susan Forsyth et al. v. Eli Lilly et al.*

Case No. 95-00185 ACK, United States District Court for the District of Hawaii.

74. *Defendants Eli Lilly and Company and Dista Product Company's Amended and Supplemental Answers to Plaintiff's First Interrogatories.* Plaintiff's exhibit number 179 in *Susan Forsyth et al. v. Eli Lilly et al.* Case No. 95-00185 ACK, United States District Court for the District of Hawaii.

75. T.P. Laughren, "Background comments for February 2, 2004 Meeting of Psychopharmacological Drugs Advisory Committee (PDAC) and Pediatric Subcommittee of the Anti-Infective Drugs Advisory Committee (Peds AC)," January 5, 2004 Memorandum, Department of Health and Human Services, Food and Drug Administration, Center for Drug Evaluation and Research.

76. R. Waters, "Drug report barred by FDA: scientist links antidepressants to suicide in kids," *San Francisco Chronicle,* February 1, 2004, p. A1; G. Harris, "Expert kept from speaking at antidepressant hearing," *The New York Times,* April 16, 2004, p. A16; E. Shogren, "FDA sat on report linking suicide, drugs," *Los Angeles Times,* April 6, 2004, p. A-13.

77. G. Harris, "F.D.A. links drugs to being suicidal," *The New York Times,* September 14, 2004, p. A1.

78. Shogren, "FDA sat on report linking suicide, drugs."

79. *PDR,* 2004, pp. 1583–94, 3413–24.

80. R. Hales, S. Yudofsky, *Essentials of Clinical Psychiatry,* 2nd Ed. (Washington, DC: American Psychiatric Publishing, 2000), p. 810; P. Tyrer, "Invited comment," *Acta Psychiatrica Scandinavica* 2000;102(6):467–8; P.M. Haddad and M. Qureshi, "Misdiagnosis of antidepressant discontinuation [withdrawal] symptoms," *Acta Psychiatrica Scandinavica* 2000;102(6):466–7; *Drug and Therapeutics Bulletin,* "Withdrawing patients from antidepressants," 1999; 37(7):49–52.

81. SmithKline Beecham [now GlaxoSmithKline], "Paxil (paroxetine): Patient Question & Answer Guide," July 1997; GlaxoSmithKline, "Generalized Anxiety Disorder," April 2001. The phrase "non-habit forming" was used in television advertisements.

82. *Pharmaceutical Litigation Reporter,* "Federal judge reverses order barring Paxil TV ads: case summary," October 30, 2002.

83. D. Willman, "NIMH staff must report payments," *Los Angeles Times,* May 19, 2004, p. A-15.

84. D. Willman, "Stealth merger: drug companies and government medical research; some of the National Institutes of Health's top scientists are also collecting paychecks and stock options from biomedical firms. Increasingly, such deals are kept secret," *Los Angeles Times,* December 3, 2003, p. A-1.

85. M. Angell, "The truth about drug companies," *New York Review of Books,* July 15, 2004, pp. 52–8; M. Angell, *The Truth About the Drug Companies: How They Deceive Us and What to Do About It* (New York: Random House, 2004).

86. G. Harris, "Drug companies seek to mend their image," *The New York Times,* July 8, 2004.
87. Glenmullen, *Prozac Backlash,* pp. 189–232.

Appendix 3. Tapering Tricyclic and Heterocyclic Antidepressants

1. J. Glenmullen, *Prozac Backlash: Overcoming the Dangers of Prozac, Zoloft, Paxil, and Other Antidepressants with Safe, Effective Alternatives* (New York: Simon & Schuster, 2000).
2. *British National Formulary,* 47th Ed. (London: British Medical Association and Royal Pharmaceutical Society of Great Britain, 2004).
3. J.G. Hardman and L.E. Limbird, Eds., *Goodman & Gilman's The Pharmacological Basis of Therapeutics,* 10th Edition (New York: McGraw-Hill, 2001), pp. 447–83.
4. *Physician's Desk Reference (PDR),* (Montvale, NJ: Thomson PDR, 2004); E.L. Barsuk, S.G. Schoonover, A.J. Gelenberg, *The Practitioner's Guide to Psychoactive Drugs,* 2nd Ed. (New York: Plenum Publishing, 1983). Barsuk's textbook was popular in the 1980s when tricyclic and heterocyclic antidepressants were the most widely prescribed antidepressants, before the introduction of SSRI antidepressants.
5. S.C. Dilsaver and J.F. Greden, "Antidepressant withdrawal phenomena," *Biological Psychiatry* 1984; 19(2):237–56.
6. Hardman and Limbird, Eds., *Goodman & Gilman's The Pharmacological Basis of Therapeutics,* pp. 447–83.
7. K. Demyttenaere and P. Haddad, "Compliance with antidepressant therapy and antidepressant discontinuation [withdrawal] symptoms," *Acta Psychiatrica Scandinavica* 2000;403:50–6.
8. S.C. Dilsaver, "Withdrawal phenomena associated with antidepressant and antipsychotic agents," *Drug Safety* 1994;10(2):103–14.
9. P. Haddad, "Newer antidepressants and the discontinuation [withdrawal] syndrome," *Journal of Clinical Psychiatry* 1997;58(suppl 7):17–21; discussion 22; M. Lejoyeux, J. Ades, I. Mourad, J. Solomon, S. Dilsaver, "Antidepressant Withdrawal Syndrome: Recognition, Prevention and Management," *CNS Drugs* 1996;4:278–92.
10. Dilsaver, "Withdrawal phenomena associated with antidepressant and antipsychotic agents."

Appendix 4. Tapering Monoamine Oxidase Inhibitor Antidepressants

1. J.G. Hardman and L.E. Limbird, Eds., *Goodman & Gilman's The Pharmacological Basis of Therapeutics,* 10th Edition (New York: McGraw-Hill, 2001), pp. 447–83.

2. Ibid.

3. S.C. Dilsaver, "Withdrawal phenomena associated with antidepressant and antipsychotic agents," *Drug Safety* 1994;10(2):103–14.

4. F. Therrien and J.S. Markowitz, "Selective serotonin reuptake inhibitors and withdrawal symptoms: a review of the literature," *Human Psychopharmacology* 1997;12:309–23.

5. D. Kasantikul, "Reversible delirium after discontinuation [withdrawal] of fluoxetine [Prozac]," *Journal of the Medical Association of Thailand* 1995;78(1): 53–4.

ACKNOWLEDGMENTS

I could not have written this book without the support of many friends, colleagues, students, patients, and family. I am especially appreciative of the support of three Harvard colleagues, psychiatrists who read each draft of the manuscript and provided invaluable input: Joshua Sparrow at Boston Children's Hospital, Elissa Kleinman at Cambridge Hospital, and Simon Lejeune at Massachusetts Institute of Technology Health Services. Early on, Thomas Moore at George Washington University Medical Center was extremely helpful in shaping the book. Because I wanted *The Antidepressant Solution* to be useful to primary care doctors, I am grateful to Hilary Worthen at Cambridge Hospital/Harvard Medical School for reading the manuscript. Kaethe Weingarten, also at Cambridge Hospital/Harvard Medical School, provided valuable input from the perspective of therapists who support patients through the process of antidepressant withdrawal.

In recent years, I have been fortunate to get to know many individuals and families who have survived severe antidepressant side effects and gone on to become national spokespeople in the effort to educate the public about them. Their dedication and public service have made it a privilege to work with them. Special thanks go to Jennifer Tierney, Tom Woodward, and Lisa Van Syckel. Special thanks also go to Vera Sharav, president of the Alliance for Human Research Protection, who works closely with the families. All of them read the manuscript of *The Antidepressant Solution* to ensure that it serves the needs of patients and families.

Indeed, an international network of patient advocates has sprung up in recent years to educate the public around the world about antidepressant side effects. Special thanks and credit go to those in the U.K.—Charles Medawar, Richard Brook, and David Healy—for their courage and dedicated public service. Special thanks also go to producer Andy Bell and journalist Shelley Jofre of the BBC program *Panorama*, whose ground-breaking investigations of the antidepressant scandal forced the British Medicines and Healthcare products Regulatory Agency (MHRA), the equivalent of the

U.S. FDA, to investigate the matter more responsibly, which in turn forced the FDA to do so.

I have had many gifted and supportive colleagues and friends in the departments of psychiatry and medicine at Harvard University Health Services and Cambridge Hospital/Harvard Medical School. Special thanks go to two senior faculty members, Alan Stone and Leon Eisenberg, for their endorsement of my earlier book *Prozac Backlash* and their long-standing support of my work. Special thanks also go to Linda Miller and Nina Masters in the department of psychiatry at Cambridge Hospital/Harvard Medical School. I also greatly appreciate Jay Burke's wise and steady stewardship of the department of psychiatry at Cambridge Hospital/Harvard Medical School, the hospital where I did my training in psychiatry and which has been my academic home base ever since. Special thanks also go to Tom Gutheil, Terry Maltsberger, and Harold Burszytajn in the Program in Psychiatry and the Law at Harvard Medical School. I am also grateful to Sherwin Nuland at the Yale School of Medicine, Candace Pert at the Georgetown University School of Medicine, and journalist John Horgan for their endorsement of *Prozac Backlash* and staunch support of the book at a time when writing about antidepressant-induced suicidality was much more controversial than it is today.

This book would not have been possible without the generosity of the many patients who agreed to my telling their stories in the public interest. Of course, their identities have been disguised to protect them.

Over the years I have had the good fortune to work with particularly challenging and stimulating students. Teaching talented students has helped me to articulate my approach to psychiatry.

I have been fortunate to have the astute counsel of my agent, Robert Lescher, who has stewarded all three of my books to publication. My editor for both *The Antidepressant Solution* and *Prozac Backlash*, Fred Hills, has been a master at helping shape my books and a true author's advocate. I am also indebted to his assistant, Kirsa Rein, and all the people at Free Press and Simon & Schuster for their skill in turning a manuscript into a finished book. I am also greatly appreciative of my assistant Stephanie's dedication to this book. She has often gone above and beyond the call of duty by putting in long hours included weekends to help me write the book.

Most of all I would like to thank my wife and children, to whom the book is dedicated. As young adults, my children—Ciara, Peter, and Michael— have taken a keen interest in the subject matter and writing of this book. Their growing awareness of the world around them has been a pleasure to watch. I am deeply appreciative of my wife Muireann's unwavering support and encouragement of my work.

INDEX

ABOUT THE AUTHOR

JOSEPH GLENMULLEN, M.D., is a clinical instructor in psychiatry at Harvard Medical School, on the staff of Harvard University Health Services, and in private practice in Harvard Square. A nationally recognized authority on antidepressant side effects, Dr. Glenmullen testified at the Federal Drug Administration hearing that resulted in the FDA's spring 2004 warning on the dangers, especially suicidal tendencies, of using these drugs. Dr. Glenmullen won the 2001 Annual Achievement Award from the American Academy for the Advancement of Medicine for his efforts in warning physicians and patients of the potential dangers of antidepressants in his widely acclaimed book *Prozac Backlash*. A graduate of Brown University and Harvard Medical School, Dr. Glenmullen lives with his wife and three children in Cambridge, Massachusetts, and can be found on the web at www.antidepressantsolution.com.